"*The Good Doctor*, by Kenneth Brigham and Michael Johns, could well be the first and last book taught in medical schools. It has broad appeal to others in health care in addition to the general public, for whom it is most obviously written—because everyone needs a good doctor. *The Good Doctor* dissects dilemmas of uncertainty in modern medical practice: factuality, statistics, and even the matter of truth itself. This book begs for thorough analysis, in the fashion of a liberal-arts seminar class (in classroom or by Zoom), at the beginning of medical studies and again before residency training."

—DAVID A. BLOOM,
Department of Urology, University of Michigan

"In *The Good Doctor*, Drs. Brigham and Johns share their insights regarding what are the characteristics to seek and to avoid when choosing a physician. Replete with illustrative stories, they share their perspectives gained through decades as practicing physicians at leading major medical institutions and their personal experiences as patients. They have combined their deep understanding of the current realities of medicine with the timeless truth that medicine is a person-to-person interaction to author this balanced and timely guide for all interested in choosing the 'right' physician."

—JAMES O. WOOLLISCROFT, MD, MACP, FRCP,
Lyle C. Roll Professor of Medicine, Professor of Internal Medicine and
Learning Health Sciences, and Dean Emeritus, University of Michigan
Medical School

"A delightful read that will challenge preconceptions and provoke critical contemplation. It will make the lay reader a better patient and informed consumer of health care and make the medical reader a better provider of health care."

—JEFF KOPLAN, MD, MPH,
Vice President for Global Health, Emory University, and former
director of the US Centers for Disease Control and Prevention

THE GOOD DOCTOR
Why Medical Uncertainty Matters

Kenneth Brigham, M.D.
and Michael M. E. Johns, M.D.

Seven Stories Press
New York • Oakland • Liverpool

Seven Stories Press
140 Watts Street
New York, NY 10013
www.sevenstories.com

Library of Congress Cataloging-in-Publication Data

Names: Brigham, Kenneth L., author. | Johns, Michael M. E., author.
Title: The good doctor / Kenneth Brigham, M.D. and Michael M.E. Johns, M.D.
Description: New York, NY : Seven Stories Press, 2020.
Identifiers: LCCN 2020008106 (print) | LCCN 2020008107 (ebook) | ISBN
  9781609809966 (hardcover) | ISBN 9781609809973 (ebook)
Subjects: LCSH: Physician and patient. | Communication in medicine. |
  Medicine--Decision making. | Uncertainty.
Classification: LCC R727.3 .B72 2020 (print) | LCC R727.3 (ebook) | DDC
  610.69/6--dc23
LC record available at https://lccn.loc.gov/2020008106
LC ebook record available at https://lccn.loc.gov/2020008107

College professors and high school and middle school teachers may order free examination copies of Seven Stories Press titles. To order, visit www.sevenstories.com, or
fax on school letterhead to (212) 226-1411.

Printed in the USA.

9 8 7 6 5 4 3 2 1

For every complex problem there is an answer that
is clear, simple, and wrong.

—H. L. MENCKEN

CONTENTS

AUTHORS' NOTE

This book is an inside job. Combined, the authors have spent a century immersed in American medicine as teachers, practitioners, researchers, administrators, and a variety of less well-defined roles. In recent years, we have also been patients with the kinds of issues that come with age and life experience, sometimes trivial and sometimes not. So, we know some things about doctors—what kinds of people they are, why they chose their profession, how they were educated, what drives them, what disappoints them about their job, how they relate to their patients and colleagues, etc.—that we think will interest anyone seeking their services and will help the medical outsider (of course that's most folks) to choose well. And we've seen health care from the other side too. For reasons that will become obvious, we think that some understanding of the human, scientific, and technical intricacies of medicine can smooth out the potential rough spots where health care happens at the interface of the profession with the people it serves.

Uncertainty plays a ubiquitous and critical role in health care, which is why we think that doctors who are too sure of almost anything can be dangerous. The best possible health care means partnering with a doctor who is intimate with uncertainty and not intimidated by it. If this emphasis on uncertainty doesn't sound as serious as the subject deserves, don't be misled. There is probably no more serious and challenging issue in all of medicine than coming to grips with this fact. In the medical world, *maybe* is a pretty serious word.

Our hope is that the reader will come away from this book with a better understanding of doctors, who they are and how and why they do what they do. And most of all, we hope that each reader emerges better prepared to identify the health care setting that is the best possible one for them (hint: they won't all be the same). That would change health care for the better and possibly save lives.

If by chance you are contemplating a medical career or are a ways down that path already, we hope the book will influence the kind of professional you strive to become.

PROLOGUE

What This Book Is About

There are a couple of critical facts about health care that a lot
of us—doctors, patients, administrators, managers, insurers,
and health systems people—don't really understand. Because
of that, we too often choose doctors for the wrong reasons,
doctors who give us less than ideal care in inefficient clinics
that are driven by the wrong motives. It doesn't have to be
that way.

One critical fact is that *uncertainty is integral to medicine.*
Uncertainty is the trigger for discovery and discovery is what
enables a new future for medicine and health care. Uncertainty also makes medical evidence pliable enough that it
can be made to fit the unique person that is each of us.

Another critical and underappreciated fact is that *your personal health care is a collaboration.* Neither you nor your doctor
can do this alone. The best possible health care involves a
partnership between two real human beings—your doctor
and you—who need to get to know each other; computers
are important and will become more so, but they will never
be able to do the whole job.

If we, that is the royal we, can understand and act on those
two basic facts, we can exploit the scary power of exploding
science and technology to make our health care better than it
has ever been. But if we ignore the vital role of uncertainty,
underestimate the value of the doctor-patient partnership,

and count on the technologists to solve the problem, we will not be pleased with the results. And you don't need the politicians and policy makers to start you on the path to good care. You can begin to nudge things in the right direction by dealing with your personal health care wisely.

This book is an attempt to explore how those two basic facts affect the kind of doctor we think you need to look for and to suggest how to go about finding and relating to such a doctor. There is also some discussion of the effects of these two facts on how new truths are discovered and communicated and how health care is perceived, organized, and carried out. After all, what medical scientists discover, what our society decides to do with those discoveries, and how new truths get translated into medical practice are the ammunition that you and your doctor have to help you take on the particular uncertainties in your personal care.

The good doctor never gets too comfortable with accepted dogma. She questions herself and everyone else from the time she begins her medical journey until she's done. But she's okay with uncertainty. In fact, that's maybe one reason she chose medicine as a profession, and it certainly explains her comfort with the essential human ambiguity that practicing medicine keeps forcing her to face. If you want to be as healthy as you can be, this is the doctor you need to get to know.

PART I

Some Basics

CHAPTER 1

The Doctor You Want (It's Not Who You Think)

Why would you entrust your health care to a doctor who is always looking for alternative explanations, questioning whether the obvious is really true, and wondering whether something important is being overlooked? When you fall ill, you feel a pretty urgent need to be told exactly what is wrong and what to do about it. You want your doctor to give you clear yes-or-no answers that you can believe and act on. After all, the doctor spent all those years learning how bodies work, what can go wrong, and when things go wrong how to get them back on track. And at least since the late nineteenth century when William Osler, the much revered godfather of modern American medicine, took over the reins at Johns Hopkins, medicine has benefitted from the rigor and genius of cutting-edge science and technology. With all of that incredible history and the consequent chain reaction of medical discovery that continues to expand, isn't it reasonable to expect your doctor to be pretty darn sure of what's causing that cramping pain in your stomach that comes and goes, sometimes waking you up at night, and to either cut it out or give you a pill that will fix it? You don't want to wait too long to see the doctor, huddled with a dozen other miserable fellow humans, thumbing through old magazines or watching repeating rounds of *Headline News* stories, just to come away with a list of possibilities. No, you want to come away with a concrete diagnosis and precise therapy. Isn't that what doctors are supposed to do for you?

Sometimes it works that way. If you have a sore throat, an earache, or fever and a cough, the odds are that you will come away from visiting your doctor with a pretty clear idea of the situation and a specific treatment plan, both of which are likely to be right for you. The same is true if you show up at a hospital emergency room drenched in sweat with crushing chest pain and a falling blood pressure. We have learned an enormous amount about human health and disease in the last century, and so most doctors are even more likely than Dr. Osler was to accurately diagnose and effectively treat a good number of human conditions. Both you and your doctor can feel pretty confident that the right things are being done when the problem is simple and straightforward.

But the problem is not always simple. Rarely that earache which seems for all the world like a run-of-the-mill middle ear infection turns out to be caused by something more serious, like a malignant tumor of the throat. It is hard to be absolutely sure of a diagnosis even when things seem pretty straightforward. In spite of all these years of accumulated knowledge, there is still a lot of uncertainty in medicine.

So who you really want for your doctor is a person who is comfortable with uncertainty, who understands that yes-or-no answers are rewarding when they are true but that sometimes the answer is neither yes nor no. You want a doctor with the courage to boldly declare that the answer is often *maybe*. When things get serious and the situation complicated, that doctor might be your best chance for continuing to reside on the living side of the great divide, where most of us would like to remain for as long as possible.

Not everyone believes that. If you want clarity and unwavering confidence, there are doctors who are more than willing to accommodate you. There is a persistent illusion of the doctor as an image of authority, keeper of the secrets of life, arbiter of proper behavior. *Doctor's orders* carry the weight of implied infallibility. But that attitude is patently contrived, misleading, counterproductive, and risky.

So if your choice is between a doctor who is absolutely sure about your condition and one who equivocates a bit, we advise choosing the latter; the other one either doesn't understand the situation or is deceiving her- or himself or you or both. It's the maybes, the universe of possibilities, in medicine that make room for dealing with the infinite variations on the theme of humanness—what Dr. Seuss calls *the you that is You*. Ambiguity is a real advantage when making life and death decisions that affect real, as opposed to statistically created, theoretical people. The doctor who is in touch with the ambiguities is likely to integrate the known facts with all of the other available information about you as a unique individual before deciding on a diagnosis and treatment; that doctor is more likely to get it right.

The good doctor's brain bristles with the vast storehouse of relevant medical knowledge, *what is*, but the door to her mind is always ajar, open to the even vaster world of *what might be*. She knows above everything else that the rapidly expanding body of medical knowledge, at its most certain, is abstract and that the reality of health care is each of the flesh-and-blood human beings patiently waiting for her help in an office exam room. She knows that we are all different, and she can approach each of us with confidence because she understands that what is known in medicine, the evidence, must be applied to each unique person in her care. She knows that how certain she can be that the available evidence fits a particular patient varies with both the nature of the evidence and the nature of the patient and that the uncertainties are where her tailoring skills can improve the fit.

Michelle Roper (not her real name) knows, from personal experience, the difference between a doctor who is satisfied with the obvious and a doctor whose mind is open to other possibilities. Ms. Roper was thirty-five years old when she showed up in the medical clinic at an elite academic medical center with a chief complaint of, "I think my lung has collapsed again." When asked what she meant by "again," she recounted that her lung had collapsed several times over the previous year, sometimes requiring that a tube be put in her chest to get the lung to re-expand. Although she had always recovered without too much trouble, she knew that a collapsed lung could be serious, even life threatening, and she really didn't like the fact that the problem kept recurring. She lived in constant fear that the next one might be fatal. Her doctor must have thought, hmm . . . it isn't too unusual for a young woman's lung to collapse once, but it shouldn't keep happening over and over . . . maybe there is more to this story.

Ms. Roper was generally in good health except that she was being treated by her gynecologist for endometriosis—a condition where small islands of tissue like that which lines the womb wind up somewhere else, usually on the lining of the abdominal cavity. At the time of menstruation, these little islands slough off some of their cells and bleed into the abdomen, often causing severe cramps.

Ms. Roper was breathing too fast and said that she had a sharp sudden pain on the right side of her chest and got suddenly short of breath several hours earlier. When asked whether she was menstruating, she said that her period had started on the previous day, but wanted to know why that was important; no one had asked her that question when her lung had collapsed before. The doctor replied that, while he had never personally seen such a case, he had read that sometimes endometriosis could implant those islands of womb tissue on the covering of the lungs. At menstruation, when the tissue sloughed off some cells, it could make a small hole in the lung that would let air leak out into the chest and cause the lung to collapse, a condition called *catamenial* (from Greek for monthly) *pneumothorax* [air (pneumo) in the chest cavity (thorax)]. After getting her lung re-expanded, Ms. Roper was treated with hormones to suppress her menses and had no further difficulty with her lungs.

When her doctor was making rounds one day while Ms. Roper was in the hospital, she volunteered, "You know, my sister says that during her periods she always gets pain in her chest and feels short of breath. I wonder if she has the same thing."

The doctor smiled, remembering William Osler's admonition to "listen to the patient; he is telling you the diagnosis." Ms. Roper's sister was asked to come to the clinic at the time of her next menstrual period, and when she did, a chest x-ray showed a partially collapsed lung. The experience resulted in a report in the literature of the only known cases of two members of the same immediate family with menses-associated lung collapse (*familial catamenial pneumothorax*).

A collapsed lung is not a rare occurrence and the reason for it is almost never found, so the accurate diagnosis is usually *spontaneous pneumothorax*. Ms. Roper's earlier doctors had the right diagnosis, pneumothorax, but they failed to recognize the distinctly rare underlying cause. Her pneumothorax was not at all spontaneous. By listening to the patient and thinking of unusual possibilities, a more inquisitive doctor discovered not only the root cause of Ms. Roper's problem, but that of her sister as well.

The myth of the infallible doctor has worn out its welcome. The traditional authoritative doctor-obedient patient arrangement no longer serves to make us healthier. The truth is that the doctor isn't always right and the patient always brings critical information. What we need is an equal partnership between the person seeking medical care and a doctor who knows and thoroughly understands the current data and as a result, has a firm grip on the uncertainties. Expectations need to change. The public and the profession should understand that uncertainty is integral to medical practice and is an essential good that allows your doctor to deal effectively with you. Maybe even save your life!

But how could uncertainty save your life? Isn't the goal of medicine to understand health and disease so thoroughly that the doctor can rely on scientifically proven facts to arrive at a certain conclusion about what you have and what to do about it? And, if we aren't quite there yet, aren't we close enough that uncertainty will be the exception rather than the rule?

The truth is that we aren't that close to eliminating medical uncertainty and will never reach that ultimate goal because each one of us is different in ways that influence our health and how we respond to disease; there are few universal truths. The next chapter explains why we believe that not only is medical uncertainty real and inescapable, but that it is also necessary for each unique one of us to benefit most from the available evidence. That is why you want the help of the good doctor.

CHAPTER 2

Uncertainty Is Essential to Personal Health Care

A middle-aged woman who worked as a laboratory technician at a major university medical center developed high blood pressure because one of her kidneys was abnormal and had to be removed. When her physician employer went to visit her after surgery, he found her barely responsive even though there had been plenty of time for the anesthesia to wear off. She lay motionless in the bed breathing about five or six times a minute, did not respond at all even when her visitor shouted directly into her ear, and barely winced when he pinched the tendon at the back of her heel, a standard test for seeing whether a patient responds to pain. The doctor looked in her chart and discovered that the eighty-five-pound woman had been given an exorbitant dose of narcotic for her age and size. He paged the resident who was responsible for the service and asked why this petite woman had been given a man-size dose of drug. The resident responded. "That's a standard post-op dose."

"But," the physician protested, "she's not a standard woman!"

No doubt the resident was right; he had given a standard post-op dose of narcotic. But standard practice almost killed his patient. The possibility that the recommended dose might not fit the specific situation just didn't cross this confident young doctor's mind and so he failed to adapt the standard to the person he was treating. If that sounds like a lapse in common sense rather than a lack of knowledge, that was probably true in this case, but it raises a larger question. How does my doctor come to a conclusion about what I have and what to do about it?

The answer to that question has two parts: What are the facts (doctors call that *evidence based medicine*)? and How do the facts fit your specific situation (doctors call that *personalized or precision medicine*)?

WHERE DO MEDICAL FACTS COME FROM?

They come from accurately analyzed research done according to scrupulous scientific principles. A lot has been learned about human health and disease from such studies and in the twenty-first century, the learning curve is steeper than it has ever been. Doctors can rely confidently on a very large and expanding store of medical facts in their efforts to help us stay healthy or get well.

Most facts that are relevant to your health come from studies done on groups of people, often very large groups. Facts from those studies are based on statistics and they are never absolute. Depending on a host of things, including size of the study, what kind of people were studied, how carefully the study was designed, and whether there is more than one study that reached the same conclusions, your doctor's confidence in the facts may vary. There is always some degree of uncertainty about the accuracy of the available information from studies with human participants; our species just isn't that predictable.

There are a number of reasons to be less than absolutely sure about medical information that comes from studies in people. Even conclusions from carefully done research may not survive the trials of time and technology. Here are two examples.

In a series of detailed studies on human volunteers done with colleagues at the Rockefeller Institute in the early 1950s, Lewis Dahl concluded that a rice and fruit diet was effective treatment for high blood pressure because the diet was low in sodium. Dr. Dahl found that he could produce high blood pressure, with all of its complications, in rats by giving them big doses of salt. He gathered data from Eskimos, Marshall Islanders, North Americans, southern Japanese, and northern Japanese and produced a lovely graph showing a nearly perfect relationship between how much salt people ate and how many had high blood pressure. The Institute of Medicine, the U.S. Food and Drug Administration, and the U.S. Senate Select Committee on Nutrition and Human Needs were so convinced by Dr. Dahl's studies that they issued an edict that we should all eat less salt if we want to be healthy and live a long and happy life—the less salt the better.

Then, an analysis of a large number of studies of the relationship between salt intake and health reported in the *American Journal of Hypertension* in April of 2014 concluded that, "Both low sodium intakes and high sodium intakes are associated with *increased* [emphasis added] mortality." The final answer about how salt intake relates to health will require some more research in this area, but what Dr. Dahl and others established as a scientific fact that drove individual behavior, medical practice, and social policy for decades may have been an oversimplification.

And there is the notion that eating fat is bad for one's heart and blood vessels. Ancel Keys, a brilliant and charismatic nutritionist, collected information about deaths from heart disease and diet in seven countries and published his results as a book in 1980. His work (and his effective advocacy) convinced the American Heart Association and the federal government to issue dietary guidelines based on his conclusion that eating fat was bad for the heart. Those events radically changed the American diet with enormous industrial, economic, and personal consequences. But an analysis of data from over half a million people from 76 different studies published in the *Annals of Internal Medicine* in 2014 concludes that "Current evidence does not clearly support cardiovascular guidelines that encourage high consumption of polyunsaturated fatty acids and low consumption of total saturated fats." That's scientific argot for eating fat doesn't cause heart disease as far as we can tell from the available data. The medical "truth" may be different than what it was in 1980.

So time and technology can change the facts. And what we believe about health is influenced by a lot of other things—opinions of prominent public personalities, promiscuous advertising, personal beliefs, societal pressures—that are not reliable sources of accurate information. Then there are the quacks looking to make a buck at your expense, entrenched cultural attitudes, and ambiguities in the discovery process that add to the uncertainties. And there is always the money magnet tugging at honest and well-meaning professionals.

If your doctor wants to practice *evidence-based medicine* (we hope so), she should have a firm grasp of what "evidence" she can be pretty sure about and when to respond to a "fact" as someone once wrote on the flyleaf of the Bible, "interesting if true."

HOW DO THE FACTS FIT YOU?

We are all members of the same species and so there is a storehouse of facts about humans that fits all of us. However, a lot of the critical evidence for these facts is based on statistics. A thinking doctor knows that statistics describe groups of people, not individuals. If she wants to practice *personalized medicine* (we hope so), she needs to figure out how the numbers describing what happens in a group of people relate to you. The statistics may not help her do that; in fact they can be misleading.

In his wonderful essay, "The Median Isn't the Message," the late Harvard paleontology professor Stephen Jay Gould makes this point. The median is one of the statisticians' favorite numbers. It is a number in the middle of the group data; by definition, half the people score above the median and half below. While still a young man, Dr. Gould got the potentially devastating news that he had abdominal mesothelioma, described to him as a fatal disease with a median survival of five months. But he wasn't ready to settle for a median fate and he knew a thing or two about statistics. He did an extensive search of the available information and discovered that while the median survival of people with abdominal mesothelioma was indeed five months and most of its victims died quickly, a few people with the disease lived much longer than the median, even years longer. After a careful look at the specifics of his own situation, Dr. Gould concluded that he was one of those lucky folks. He lived for another twenty years, eventually dying of something else. Statistical conclusions from even the most rigorously done population studies may be irrelevant to you and may lead you down a path to either despair or confidence with no good reason for either.

Rigorously done and carefully analyzed studies in groups of people with a given condition will always be essential "evidence" informing efforts to figure out what you have and what should be done about it. But the value of such evidence depends on both how well the studies were done and how relevant they are to your specific circumstance. The wise doctor pays careful attention to the numbers, but she is not mesmerized by them. Numbers are not indisputable and unique criteria for personal health related decisions. *Evidence is absolutely necessary but not always sufficient.* That's why we need uncertain doctors.

RECONCILING EVIDENCE-BASED AND PERSONALIZED HEALTH CARE

You want a doctor who is comfortable with uncertainty because what she doesn't know could save your life. How much liberty your doctor dare take in bending the evidence to suit your particular situation depends on what evidence there is and how sure your doctor is that it is true and rel-

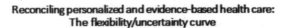

Reconciling personalized and evidence-based health care: The flexibility/uncertainty curve

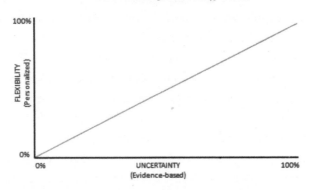

evant to you (that is, how much she doesn't know). This relationship between relying on the evidence and taking into account the idiosyncratic you in arriving at a diagnosis and therapy can be illustrated by a simple graph. How much your doctor can justify modifying her approach to diagnosis and treatment because you don't exactly fit the usual mold (*flexibility*) is directly related to what she doesn't know, that is, how *uncertain* she is about the available evidence. If there were evidence that was 100 percent certain to be true for every human being (0 percent uncertainty), then there would be no need to massage the program to suit a specific person. It would truly be a one-size-fits-all solution. You wouldn't even need a doctor in that case. You could just look it up on the internet.

Of course, in human biology there is no such animal, but for some situations there is excellent evidence in many different kinds of people so it is pretty clear what to do. The need for a personalized approach is not so great in that case; there is a good chance that any one of us will do well on the same evidence-based treatment. As the evidence becomes less certain, the need and the opportunity for fitting the intervention to the specific person being treated increases. Where there is no credible evidence (100 percent uncertainty), your doctor and you are on your own. In that situation, individual preferences, specific experiences, anecdotes, knowledgeable opinions, and personal priorities might help determine what to do and those decisions are unconstrained by "evidence." It's up to your doctor and you to do the best you can with whatever information you can get your hands on.

So one source of the good doctor's uncertainty is whether a treatment that usually works in large groups of people will work for you. But that assumes that there is no doubt about what she is trying to treat, that she is sure about the diagnosis. What if the evidence for a specific diagnosis is not so clear? That is not an unusual situation. Arriving at a diagnosis is sometimes a journey rather than an event. The journey follows the pattern illustrated in the graph, progressing down the slope of decreasing uncertainty until finally arriving at the origin with an unequivocal diagnosis; therapy may be different at different points along the journey.

Here is an example. About every six weeks over sixteen months a forty-four-year-old man had three or four days of fever, aching in his arms and legs, and drenching sweats at night. Between those episodes he felt fine. His general physician could find nothing wrong on a physical exam and a battery of lab tests was normal. When he reappeared five months later with more frequent episodes, he was referred for a second opinion. Infectious disease experts noted that he now had pain in his leg and shoulder joints, but again physical and extensive lab examinations were all normal. With nothing specific to go on, his doctors thought he might have some obscure infection or an autoimmune disease. Someone suggested the possibility of an immune system related disorder called Still's disease. After seven more months, the patient was sent to an academic rheumatology unit where nothing specific was discovered. However, the working diagnosis was Still's disease and he was treated initially with a non-steroidal anti-inflammatory agent (NSAID). When he didn't improve, he was given a corticosteroid and methotrexate, potent medicines for immune related disorders like Still's disease. In spite of the potent medicines, the patient gradually developed obvious arthritis in his joints and some abnormal non-specific lab tests. Finally, almost six years after his initial vague complaints caused him to seek help from his general doctor, the patient developed frequent watery diarrhea and rapid weight loss. At that point, a biopsy of his small intestine revealed the classical findings of a rare disease of the intestine first described by George Whipple in 1907 and subsequently shown to be due to an infection with an unusual bacterium. Whipple's disease is often associated with arthritis but diarrhea and weight loss are the essential clues to the diagnosis.

So for six years, this unfortunate patient endured a long and difficult journey down the path toward less and less uncertainty through several possible diagnoses and several unsuccessful therapies, to finally arrive at a clear diagnosis.

Now how about therapy?

Treatment of Whipple's disease involves a year course of antibiotics, but which antibiotics? Therapy of rare diseases is fraught with uncertainty. There are too few cases of Whipple's disease to do careful trials of different antibiotics, so a regimen has to be designed based on less than stellar evidence. How to go about that?

Here's what a thinking doctor would do. She would sit down with the patient and review the efficacy, side effects, and complications of the various regimens that have been used. How many patients have a good initial response? What is the relapse rate? What is the cost to the patient? How many pills must be taken and how often? Does the patient have any allergies? Has he taken antibiotics in the past and if so were there any complications or unpleasant side effects? Taking all of those things into account, she and the patient would design an individual-specific treatment regimen based on the best evidence available, given the inherent level of uncertainty. She would closely monitor whether the patient's response to this carefully designed regimen was positive, negative, or equivocal. Depending on his response, she would move him up or down the uncertainty-flexibility curve shown in the figure and that would determine his continuing therapy. Toeing that fine line that relates the evidence to a specific person demands the skill of an experienced professional. That's why it matters so much who you choose for your doctor.

WON'T A COMPLETE ANALYSIS OF YOUR GENOME ELIMINATE UNCERTAINTY?

Some knowledgeable people would go even further and ask: *With the complete analysis of my genome in hand, why will I need a doctor at all?* And there are some impressive anecdotes that tempt us to think that perhaps we should be hunting for a good geneticist or a more powerful computer to take over responsibility for our health care instead of looking for the right doctor.

Writing in the *New York Times*, Gina Kolata introduces one of those impressive anecdotes in the person of Dr. Lukas Wartman. Dr. Wartman got interested in leukemia as a medical student. He was gearing up for a career doing research in that area when, during his last year of med school, ironically, he developed the disease himself. Chemotherapy suppressed his cancer for a while and when it recurred, a bone marrow transplant seemed effective for a bit. By then he was an assistant professor on the faculty of Washington University in Saint Louis, an amiable colleague of the excellent scientists at that institution. His leukemia came back yet again. Survival after two recurrences of his kind of leukemia is so rare that there are no statistics. There was no known treatment for his disease at that point and his health was rapidly heading south.

Dr. Wartman's genetics colleagues decided that they were not going to lose their associate without a serious fight. For the first time ever, they mapped out the entire complement of genes and measured their activity in Dr. Wartman's leukemic cells and in his normal cells and compared the two results. "Eureka!" Archimedes would have shouted. They found a gene that was going gangbusters and its product was a stimulator of the leukemic cells. What's more (eureka! again), there was a drug that was known to switch off that gene, although it had only been used to treat kidney cancer. Dr. Wartman took the drug and, for all practical purposes, got well (the appropriately cautious cancer doctors would say that he went into remission). He also had another bone marrow transplant in case his cancer developed resistance to the drug. Dr. Wartman remained in remission at least for several months, remains apparently well three or so years after the *precise* treatment of his cancer.

Hoping that experiences like Dr. Wartman's can be scaled up, the National Cancer Institute has begun enrolling thousands of patients with intractable cancers from 2,400 clinics scattered across the country. Their cancers' genomes will be analyzed and they will be given anti-cancer drugs that the genetics predict might be effective. This is an entirely new way to match therapy to the essential nature of the disease (the institute has named the study the MATCH trial). And, no doubt, this is just the beginning. The technology is irresistible. It is virtually certain that genetics will change how we think about and how we treat some cancers.

However, before getting too enthralled with the potential of genetics as the ultimate in personalized care, we should remember that probably only about thirty percent of our risk for the diseases we are most likely to get is explained by genetics. A critical doctor knows that and is a little less enthusiastic than President Bill Clinton and National Institutions of Health Director Francis Collins, who promised in the year 2000 that knowing the sequence of the human genome "would revolutionize the diagnosis, prevention, and treatment of most, if not all, human diseases," accomplishing "a complete transformation in therapeutic medicine." Twenty years later, we still have a way to go.

Genetics has already helped us understand our biology in new ways and will help to advance our health care as well. But for most common human diseases, the answer just isn't that simple; multiple genes are usually involved, many factors influence what a gene does other than the sequence of bases in the DNA, and in many cases, genetic risk is a minor contributor to actual risk. As with a lot of things in medicine, the thoughtful doctor's attitude toward the promise of genetics is cautious optimism.

Some would argue not only that genetics is not the final answer to fitting health care to a specific person, but that personalized medicine doesn't require genetics at all, that conscientious doctors have in fact been doing it for four hundred years. University of California, San Francisco professor of medicine John Murray complains in the *American Journal of Respiratory and Critical Care Medicine* that the definition of personalized medicine as "an emerging practice . . . that uses an individual's genetic profile to guide decisions made in regard to the prevention, diagnosis, and treatment of disease" is a blatant effort to hijack a term that describes what doctors have been doing for centuries.

The height of most doctors' dudgeon may not reach that of Dr. Murray's, but it does seem unlikely that genome sequences, no matter how complete, affordable, and available, will ever tell the whole story. Important parts of the story are not written in what NIH Director Francis Collins calls the "language of life."

What doctors don't know nourishes discoveries that advance medicine. And it is also the uncertainties, those niggling ambiguities, that give your doctor and you the latitude to tailor the evidence-based dogma to fit your unique case.

CHAPTER 3

Finding Your Doctor: A Field Guide

Your pool of potential personal doctors may be limited for a number of reasons—insurer, health system, geography, availability, etc. However, almost any health care insurance allows you some say in choosing a primary care doctor. This needs to be a personal relationship, and so you don't want to settle for a default doctor if you can possibly avoid it. Of course there are no perfect doctors since they, like the rest of us, are human beings. But you're not looking for perfection. What is most important if you are to be as healthy as you can be is not your doctor's perfection, but whether this specific doctor-patient partnership is going to work for you over the long haul.

Predicting the course of relationships is always a hazardous business, but if you pay attention early on, you can improve your chances of making this partnership at least functional. Start by paying careful attention to your personal feelings about encounters with the doctor. After a first visit or two, reflect on the experience, ask yourself a few questions and answer them as honestly as possible: Are you convinced that this doctor tells you the truth . . . the whole story? Are you convinced that she not only listens to you but hears what you're saying? Are you comfortable revealing to her everything about yourself that could be in any way related to your health? Are you reasonably comfortable in her presence naked (or nearly so)? Do you believe that she is genuinely interested in you as a fellow human being? Does she seem happy with her job? There is also your gut reaction to the situation that should not be ignored even if it is difficult to be specific about. What did this visit really feel like? Would you hesitate to return to this doctor when you need to?

The goal in this hunt is to find a doctor who doesn't just know what she is doing but who cares for those for whom she is doing it. Here are some observations and suggestions that may help to identify the best doctor for you from among the possible choices.

1. *You want a doctor who listens*, preferably for longer than eighteen seconds; that's how long the average doctor is said to listen to a patient before interrupting. In his book, *How Doctors Think*, Harvard physician Jerome Groopman claims that doctors don't just interrupt the patient's story after eighteen seconds, they also make snap judgments about a diagnosis at that point and tend to fixate on that judgment. And they're often wrong; somewhere between 15 and 25 percent of patients are misdiagnosed. After all, you can't tell the doctor your diagnosis, as Osler says you will, unless the doctor listens to you. It may be easier to order a bunch of tests than to listen to your story, but it is less efficient and more likely to miss something important. It also runs up the cost.

The very fact that a history of the present illness has always been considered a critical part of the doctor-patient encounter and of the medical record implies that the patient tells a story and the doctor listens to it. But even if your doctor resists the eighteen-second urge to interrupt, she may not be listening. Hearing and listening are not the same; they use different parts of the brain. Most people are not good listeners. When adults sit through a ten-minute oral presentation, half of them can't describe what they heard after only a few minutes and three fourths can't do it forty-eight hours later.

Listening skills have not been a prominent part of medical education until recently. However, professional and commercial health care organizations, motivated by accumulating evidence that listening doctors' patients are healthier, are making efforts to improve physicians' listening skills. Apparently those skills can be taught, and the results are better patient outcomes and happier and more efficient doctors.

There may be some nature as well as nurture operating here. The composer Aaron Copland, whose livelihood depended on listeners, said that listening was a gift, an "inborn talent of some degree." Granted the gift "can be trained and developed," and efforts to do that are laudable, but perhaps you should look for a doctor who is an instinctive listener, who has the gift, who knows in her bones that the chief complaint is yours not hers and so pays careful attention to what you have to say. You will recognize this person on your first visit. She will listen to you for longer than eighteen seconds, probably a lot longer.

"The ideal listener, it seems to me," Copland writes, "would combine the preparation of the trained professional with the innocence of the intuitive amateur." We like that. We want doctors with the deep knowledge and broad understanding of medicine and of human nature of "a trained professional," but who listen to our story free of bias and snap judgments, "with the innocence of the intuitive amateur."

2. You want a doctor who recognizes black swans. In his book, *The Black Swan*, Nassim Nicholas Taleb uses the metaphor to mean discoveries that are not predictable and have a large impact on what we know (before the first black swan was discovered, all swans were white). So you want your doctor to be always alert to unexpected information that upsets conventional thinking. She does not dismiss outliers out of hand, but ponders what they could mean. She stays aware of research in medicine and related areas and, while suspicious of the hype, looks carefully for tidbits that may have big implications. She does that with your personal information as well. Is there something in your story or in the test results that doesn't exactly jibe, and is that a clue that your case is due for a thorough re-examination?

3. You want a doctor who sees the gorilla. The reference is to maybe the best-known experiment in human psychology. If you aren't familiar with the experiment, you should stop reading this book, get on the internet, go to www.theinvisiblegorilla.com/gorilla_experiment.html and watch the video.

While at Harvard, psychologists Christopher Chabris and Daniel Simmons made the video of two teams of people with different color shirts passing a basketball around. The observer is charged with counting the number of times one of the teams passes the ball. In the middle of the video, a person in a gorilla suit walks to the center of the screen, thumps his chest and walks off after about nine seconds. When Chabris and Simmons had Harvard students watch the video and count the number of passes, fully half of the students got the number of passes right, but did not see the gorilla. The behavioral principle operating here is that we see what we are focused on to the exclusion of even major events outside our area of focus.

You want a doctor who both counts the number of passes of the basketball accurately and sees the gorilla. That is, she is thoroughly aware of the obvious and expected information, but not so fixated on it that something important but unexpected is missed. She is not so satisfied with establishing a diagnosis and a treatment plan that her mind is closed to other possibilities. Your health care and treatment are processes, not events. This is an enduring partnership with you at its center. Your doctor's knowledge of who you are lets her see the unexpected incongruities that are tipoffs that something is amiss.

4. You want a doctor who hears the hoof beats of zebras. The universal admonition to medical students, "When you hear hoof beats, think horses, not zebras," was apparently coined in the late 1940s by Theodore Woodward, University of Maryland infectious disease specialist and medical department chairman. It has been used ever since as a diagnostic metaphor for the truism, common things are common. Our good doctor has heard that old saw all of her professional life, but she isn't as taken with it as she once was. She also learned from Johns Hopkins professor of medicine A. McGehee Harvey that "In making the diagnosis of the cause of illness in an individual case, calculations of probability have no meaning." For a solitary person, those hoof beats are just as likely to come from zebras as horses. Sometimes doctors go through major intellectual contortions trying to turn zebras into horses and cause a lot of difficulty for their patients and themselves in the process.

Nancy Pogue's (not her real name) personal experience is a good example. Ms. Pogue spent fourteen years seeing a number of doctors about her joint weakness, pain and eventually a fluctuating blood pressure. She was told at various times that she might have multiple sclerosis, lupus, irritable bowel syndrome, or fibromyalgia. Finally, she saw a new doctor and introduced herself by declaring, somewhat defensively, that she was not a hypochondriac, something was really wrong. Sensing that Ms. Pogue's past encounters with medicine had been less than satisfactory, the doctor responded, "Try me." Then the doctor proceeded to listen attentively to Ms. Pogue's symptoms and ask a lot of questions that Ms. Pogue did not see as relevant. After pondering the history and examining Ms. Pogue's skin and joints the doctor, for the first time in the fourteen-year history of this patient's illness, arrived at the correct diagnosis of Ehler-Danlos syndrome, a congenital disease of connective tissue that can present in many different ways. Patients with this disease sometimes even refer to themselves as medical zebras.

Ironically, Dr. Woodward's axiom is less and less relevant even to his specialty, infectious diseases, as global travel becomes increasingly common. The most likely explanation of bloody urine in a young woman who has spent her life in Minnesota is a urinary tract infection. But for a young woman who moved to Minnesota three years earlier from a refugee camp in Kenya, the most likely cause is schistosomiasis, a disease virtually never seen in lifelong U.S. residents.

Horses aren't always the most likely source of hoof beats anymore—no matter where they're heard.

5. You want a doctor who is not afraid to say: I'm sorry. I was wrong. I don't know. I need help. Those are the four sentences that mystery writer Louise Penny's fictional Montreal detective Armand Gamache drums into his mentees. You want a doctor who knows those sentences and doesn't hesitate to use them. Don't buy the infallible doctor myth and avoid anyone who tries to sell you on it. This is not just an annoying pet peeve. Arrogance is a near fatal flaw in a profession that is rife with a wonderful ambiguity that enables the care of each quirky one of us. Facts are important, but don't get too fond of them; they may not be there when you need them. You want a confident doctor but not an arrogant one. Arrogance doesn't know that it doesn't know.

6. You want a doctor who doesn't overestimate the power of your genome. (You may need to hurry; the supply is rapidly dwindling.) Genomics is beginning to contribute to health care and that will only increase, but you are more than the sequence of bases in your DNA. No matter what appears in the newspapers and regardless of how many books appear on genomic medicine, you are not best served by delegating your health care to a geneticist, as important as they are. Your doctor should be thoroughly conversant with human genetics and up to date on the available tests and what they mean, but she should keep a healthy skepticism—hold on to her sense of maybe.

7. You want a doctor whom you trust, not necessarily one you like. It is very popular these days for institutions to gather information about how satisfied patients say they are with their doctors and tout that as a good reason for choosing them. The most common tool is a questionnaire that results in a Press Ganey score of patient satisfaction in a number of areas. You shouldn't pay too much attention to these scores. What you want is a doctor whom you trust, who knows her business, who *gets* the relationship between evidence-based and personalized health care, and who is honest and reliable.

There are many factors that influence Press Ganey scores. An emergency room doctor claims he got bad scores because he refused to prescribe narcotics to addicts; that might well be true. Researchers at the University of California Davis claim that "the most satisfied patients are 12 percent more likely to be hospitalized and 26 percent more likely to die." At least as currently done, attempts to equate objective scores of patient satisfaction with physician quality may be over-rated. William Sonnenberg, President of the Pennsylvania Academy of Family Physicians, writes in a Medscape article, "We can over-treat and over-prescribe. The patients will be happy, give us good ratings, yet be worse off." Your doctor must treat you with dignity and respect, but integrity and competence may have little to do with charm.

Of course you need to be aware that doctors are subject to the same maladies that afflict the rest of us—personality disorders, mental illness, depression, substance abuse, etc.—and the last thing you need is a doctor with serious behavioral issues. But, apart from confirming that a doctor is not an addict, is in reasonably good mental health, is appropriately trained, licensed, and credentialed, and has not been convicted of insurance fraud, of padding his personal bank account by doing unnecessary procedures, or of committing some heinous crime like assault or murder, we don't know of a reliable objective test of trustworthiness.

However, we are sure that a fundamental requirement is honesty. The good doctor will not always be right. She will make mistakes, possibly serious ones, but she will come clean about what is happening even when it hurts. And, of course, the mutual trust that is essential to this relationship means that you must come clean with her, even when the truth doesn't speak so well of you. You should say what you're feeling, even when you think the doctor's wrong or she displeases you. You may learn something important about the doctor from her reaction to criticism; if it's anger, be wary.

Eventually, you just have to go with your feelings about the trust thing. And first reactions can be wrong. If something seems a bit off, give the relationship a little time. If you still can't trust this doctor, you may want to look elsewhere.

Then there are the doctors to be wary of. A few examples are discussed in detail in the next section of the book. Others might include "Dr. Avatar," the robotic doctor who practices medicine by rote and has difficulty connecting with real people. You'd do well to also keep an eye out for ones who might be aptly labelled something like Dr. Hype, Dr. Dolt, or Dr. Smarm. But you should also keep in mind that if you look hard enough you'll find examples of most human personality types in the medical profession. After all, doctors are human beings, and if you expect them to be otherwise, you're in for a real disappointment. So, carefully scrutinize candidates for your personal doctor and choose the partner who works best for you.

Once you've settled on a doctor, the two of you become health care partners, collaborators in the effort to make and keep you healthy. Tell your doctor who you are, every relevant detail. She needs to know as much as possible about you to do her best job. But keep a healthy emotional distance. If you start to feel inclined to push this relationship beyond appropriate professional boundaries, or if you sense that from your doctor, back off, put some space between you. This relationship may have its obligatory intimacies, but it is not a romance. The boundaries need to be clear and respected. *Do not fall in love with your doctor* is good medical and good emotional advice. This doesn't need to be a friendship. You are professional partners, collaborators, and you need to keep the goal of this relationship—your health—in clear focus. While there must be confidence, respect, and trust on both sides, there also must be "spaces in your togetherness."

But if this is a partnership, then don't both partners share responsibility for how it works or fails to work? Do you just have to take the list of doctors you are given by whatever health care system you are in at face value and then work your way through the available options until you find somebody who seems compatible?

Maybe not. Perhaps there is something you can do to improve your chances of developing the health care relationship you're looking for. Perhaps you can help create the kind of doctor you are looking for. It might help you to do that if you had a better idea of how your doctor got to where she is and why she chose to do something that's so difficult.

CHAPTER 4

Where Doctors Come From

Some knowledge of how your doctor got to where she is might help you to understand how best to connect with her. She spent four years in college, another four in medical school, and several years of on-the-job training (internships, residencies, and fellowships) after that. Those years aimed to accomplish two things: mastery of a large body of knowledge about how the human body is put together, how it works, what can go wrong with it, and what to do when things go awry; and mastery of a set of physical and mental skills that are necessary to translate that knowledge into caring for the health of real people. All that time was devoted to accomplishing those two goals. There was not a lot of room during those years to pursue other interests in any depth. Virtually all of aspiring doctors' energies during their training are dedicated to climbing a very steep learning curve over a very long time.

If it's that hard, why would a bright young person with many options for a productive, useful, and lucrative career that would require less preparation choose to enter medicine? The almost universal answer is because they want to do something tangible, hands-on, that benefits their fellow human beings. A concern for people and a desire to do something to help others may sound like a rehearsed answer to an interviewer's question to a medical school applicant, but, trite as it sounds, that really is why most people choose a medical career. However, by the time they have clawed their way up the learning curve and are ready to start practicing medicine for real, a lot of them discover deficiencies in the unique interpersonal skills that they need to do their best, and also feel the pressures of a system that drives them in another direction. That combination—inadequate skills in the art of medicine and a system that values quantity over quality of care—can be a death knell for even the most well-intentioned doctor.

After spending all those years struggling up that daunting learning curve to the pinnacle and being granted the requisite credentials, how could a well-educated doctor, upon coming face to face with a flesh-and-blood patient, possibly feel ill-prepared for the job? Because most medical education, even now, gives pretty short shrift to the importance of dealing with that universal characteristic of flesh and blood human beings—ambiguity. There is so much other stuff to learn and such powerful history forcing medicine toward a solid footing in hard science, that the role of humanity generally takes a back seat. Many medical educators aren't very enamored of equivocal answers, i.e. *maybes*. They feel pretty good about having done their job if they can teach their charges the yeses and noes.

Almost seven decades ago, social psychologist Else Frenkel-Brunswik described *aversion to ambiguity* as a personality trait of people who are threatened by "novel, complex, or insoluble" situations. These people tend to play down or even deny ambiguity when faced with it. When confronting ambiguity that they cannot deny, these folks get seriously stressed. If there ever was a profession that requires dealing with "novel, complex, or insoluble" situations, it is clinical medicine. Medicine is rife with ambiguity and the last thing you want when you have to deal with it personally is a stressed out doctor. According to Johns Hopkins professor of medicine Gail Geller, doctors with low tolerance for ambiguity order more tests, are less likely to follow evidence-based guidelines, cost more, are more frightened of malpractice litigation, practice more defensive medicine, and are uncomfortable with death and grief. That doesn't sound like the person I need when I get sick!

But is it possible to teach people how to handle ambiguity? In other words, are doctors who deal constructively with uncertainty born, or can they be made? Is it that one comes into the world that way or not and that discomfort with uncertainty is an advantage when competing for a spot in medical school? Is it that more congenital *"antiambiguists"* enter the medical pipeline while the congenital *"ambiguists"* rejected by medical school (or discouraged from even applying), wind up doing social work or entering the ministry? Or could something be done in the process of choosing medical students and equipping them to practice medicine that would increase one's chances of locating an ambiguity-tolerant doctor? Can the pool of this kind of doctor be expanded?

Well, it could be recognized that medical students with high or low tolerance for ambiguity differ from one another in some important ways. Some studies suggest that highly tolerant students are more likely to be leaders and are more willing to practice in underserved areas. Conversely, students who are ambiguity averse are said to be more afraid of making mistakes, to have more negative attitudes toward the socially disadvantaged, and to be less tolerant of alcohol abusers. So there are clues even early in their education that attitudes toward ambiguity might affect what kind of doctors these med students are likely to become, but, at least until recently, little attention has been paid to this personality trait in either the selection of students or in the medical curriculum. Instead medical education and the culture of medicine in general have usually rewarded certainty.

There are validated scales for measuring how well one deals with ambiguity, so this factor could be considered in selecting students for medical school. In recent years, a lot of thought has been directed at whether the traditional criteria for med school admission actually choose the people who are most likely to make the best doctors. Changes in premed course requirements and in the medical college admission test (MCAT) that emphasize more humanistic qualities have been proposed and, in some cases, implemented. Time will tell whether more admission committees will start selecting students who learn the facts, understand what they are doing and why, but are more likely to embrace the essential ambiguity of human beings and to be aware of the uncertainties.

One approach to creating doctors who are more intellectually flexible is to focus specifically on teaching empathy. Massachusetts General Hospital (MGH) psychiatrist Helen Riess claims that "Empathy training enhances relationships, increases job satisfaction and improves patient outcomes." Dr. Reiss directs the MGH Empathy and Relational Science Program. She recognizes that doctors may not bring either innate or learned empathetic skills to their chosen profession, but she is convinced that adult professionals can be taught empathy. And she claims impressive results—improved outcomes with patients with diabetes, asthma, high blood pressure, obesity, and arthritis—and happier doctors.

Some medical school curricula now include teaching healthy attitudes toward uncertainty and ambiguity, but there is not much data on how effective those efforts are. There is some evidence, however, that time and experience can increase medical residents' tolerance of ambiguity. It seems likely, as with most complex personality traits, that attitudes toward ambiguity are both innate and learned. Attempts to tilt the selection and the education processes in a direction that gives the best chance to generate more contemplative doctors are laudable. It will take time and more data to know for sure if these efforts are working.

So this stern-faced and slightly disheveled person in the white coat with a stethoscope slung rakishly about her neck who strides into the exam room, asks you a bunch of highly personal questions, and has you take off your clothes, didn't just fall off the turnip truck. She's paid some dues. She's studied hard and long, seen a lot of human misery, developed a cadre of enviable technical skills, and dealt with her own life, perhaps even with personal illness. And she's had maybe a course and a couple of tutoring sessions on various aspects of the art of medicine during her training. But she is hounded by a practice manager who's not really into the soft stuff and constantly prods her to see more patients and spend less time at it. In spite of that, she continues to harbor a real love for her chosen profession. Still lurking in a warm, cozy, and passionately nurtured corner of her brain, lives the original reason she chose medicine. She really does love people and wants to do something tangible to help her patients to be healthy and happy.

Is there anything you can do to tap into that kernel of empathy, arouse that appreciation for the soft side of medicine? Can you help a doctor, struggling against the constraints of a largely dollar-driven health care system, emerge into the professional she originally dreamed of being?

But wait. Why should the doctor's professional development be your responsibility? You're paying for a service. Some would claim that you are buying health care, a product, that this is a retail transaction like buying food at the supermarket. It's not your job to do the caring; that's the doctor's job!

That is just not true. You do not buy either health or treatment of your disease at the doctor's office; if you think so, your care is not as good as it should be. Health care at its best is not a commodity; it is a partnership, a collaboration. There is an art to being a patient as well as to being a doctor, and if you don't pay some attention to your responsibilities in this relationship, as is generally true of relationships, things won't go as well as they could. The doctor may have the lion's share of the responsibility here, but you, not the doctor, will be the one who suffers most if things don't go well.

You are certainly bound by the courtesies common to relationships in general: keep appointments; show up on time; bring whatever information or medicines were asked for when you made the appointment; and have your insurance or other required information handy. And, while you should expect the doctor to spend as much time with you as is necessary to deal thoroughly with your problem, you do need to realize that there are other patients to be dealt with and that the doctor has an entire life that doesn't involve you.

You should most definitely not take a cue from Daisy Brown (not her real name). Ms. Brown was a woman in her sixties with a chronic lung problem that wasn't curable, but was well-controlled. At some point, she convinced the doctor who had cared for her for several years to take on the care of her son (in his thirties) who had asthma. At two o'clock one Monday morning, the doctor was notified that Ms. Brown's son was in the emergency room with an acute asthma attack. As the doctor was getting dressed to drive to the ER, his phone rang again. When he answered the phone, he was greeted with Ms. Brown's voice: "Doctor, since you're going to the hospital now anyway and I have an appointment to see you tomorrow afternoon, can I just come in with my son so you can see me now and save me the trip tomorrow?" The doctor suggested to Ms. Brown, in as civil a tone as he could manage, that she should keep her appointment the next afternoon. Such total disregard for the doctor's life will not do anything to enhance the quality of the medical care relationship. Even the most dedicated doctor may have had trouble resisting an inappropriate reaction to Ms. Brown's unreasonable 2:00 a.m. request.

There are some other specific things you can do to help make this relationship as good as it can be. Be clear and precise about the reason for your visit (this may take some thought); if there are several reasons, do your best to prioritize them. Make notes to help you remember everything important to tell the doctor. Even if not asked, you need to tell the doctor not only what your physical complaint(s) is but also what concerns you most about it. Whether you are most frightened about possible surgery or worried about getting day care for your kids, or about transportation to the clinic, or any of countless other possible concerns, can make a lot of difference to how your physical complaint is best dealt with. And you need to be sure that you leave the visit with an accurate understanding of the information and instructions the doctor has shared with you; ask questions and tell the doctor when you don't understand.

Then there is a basic responsibility to be totally honest with your doctor. That includes clearly saying what you feel about the experience, good or bad. There is a lot of evidence that doctors give the best care when they feel good about what they are doing, feel that they have done a good job. That is often more important than how much money they make. Your explicit appreciation for what feels like a job well done will pay off in the quality of your care. Conversely, if you don't tell the doctor that you're not happy with your care and why or that you disagree with the plan for whatever reasons, how will she know how to better meet her responsibility? Keep in mind that she is there, showing up every day to face needy people, because of that kernel of empathy that may be struggling against the constraints of the system, and that your heartfelt appreciation of her efforts could have a big effect on how good your health care is likely to be. This is a partnership.

In spite of your best efforts, it still might not work out. You may encounter a doctor whose potential for being the kind of doctor you need never existed in the first place (as we said earlier, that is a minority, but there are some); whose last kernel of empathy has succumbed to the burdens of a system that undervalues caring, uncertainty, and personal commitment; or whose noble motives have been overwhelmed by the money magnet. Aah, that devilish money magnet!

University of California, San Francisco physician Timothy Judson and University of Pennsylvania behavioral economist Kevin Volpp discuss the roles of extrinsic (read money) and intrinsic (read feeling good about one's work) motivations in affecting how doctors behave. They call one of their four scenarios *intrinsic motivation crowded out by extrinsic motivation*. In the scenario a doctor is driven by a desire to care for patients with AIDS to pursue a specialty in infectious diseases. He develops a busy practice in that area and feels really satisfied with the good he is doing for his patients. He is making a difference in their lives, and that is why he chose a medical career. He practices this way for several satisfying years. Then he discovers that doctors with less training than he had, just completing a residency in Internal Medicine, start out making more money as hospitalists than he is making after several years practicing a subspecialty. And they work only in the hospital and have designated hours. The doctor gives up the practice he loves and takes a hospitalist job for the money. Sad story, but it happens. We'd bet he's not as happy as he was.

In the following chapters, we discuss in more detail some doctors' behaviors to be wary of. You best recognize those behaviors early on and if they persist, you should probably look elsewhere for your care. However, having encountered such a physician and having decided to look elsewhere, the basic requirement for honesty demands that you say so. The same is true if you visit a different doctor, even if you return to the original one. There is the practical matter of sharing any information (tests, history, medicines, etc.) among the doctors who are caring for you, as well as the ethical demand that you come clean about what you are doing about your health care. Even a seemingly incorrigible doctor may learn something from your experience. If not, at least you tried.

So, your doctor should approach your care fully aware of and completely comfortable with the ambiguity that is inherent in your condition as a human being. The persisting kernel of empathy that still motivates her will respond to your behavior as a responsible patient. But, if this collaboration is to keep you as healthy and happy as possible, there has to be more to it. There is the potential for a mixed message as we advocate practicing evidence-based medicine while stressing how important it is to tolerate ambiguity. What is ambiguous about a practice that is driven by the evidence? Well, two things must be obvious by now: the evidence, even when it exists, may be ambiguous; and applying the evidence to a single unique individual (i.e. you) is never as simple as looking it up on the internet. There is still a lot that neither you nor your doctor knows. Things will go much better if you get that fact on the table.

In 2014, TEDMED (the branch of TED talks dealing specifically with medicine) convened to discuss "Why physicians should admit what they don't know." A couple of quotes from that program bear repeating.

Elizabeth Nabel, a cardiologist who is now president of

Boston's Brigham and Women's hospital, admonished doctors to "Have the courage to say, 'I don't know,' because it's empowering. And only then can you add, 'I'm going to find out.'"

Geneticist and director of Baylor University's Center for Medical Ethics and Health Policy Amy McGuire marveled at the power of genetics to give you the code to your existence, but recognized that not all of the answers are there. "There is no genome for the human spirit," she said.

Thinkers have recognized forever how thoroughly ambiguity permeates the human condition. "Nothing in life is certain," mused Ben Franklin, "except death and taxes." Scottish poet Robert Burns says, "There is no such uncertainty as a sure thing."

We could fill the book with quotes of this sort that are as relevant to medicine as to other life experiences. A thoughtful doctor knows that. But let's look more closely at some doctors who don't. Recognizing them could save us some time and trouble.

PART II

A Few Doctors' Maladies to Watch For

. . . And Why

CHAPTER 5

The Yes-or-No Obsession

There is no gray zone in this doctor's medical world; she deals exclusively in black and white. An unexplained abnormal test result or physical finding just drives this doctor crazy. There has to be an explanation and, by damn, she'll find it no matter what it takes. She either doesn't know or doesn't care that abnormal test results and physical findings can mean very different things in different people. This doc is a pretty concrete thinker—she doesn't truck much with individual idiosyncrasies.

The normal range of values for a test is a statistical definition; the usual boundaries are the 95 percent confidence limits. That means that five percent of normal people will have a lab test number that is defined as abnormal. But you will be wasting your time to try to convince this doctor that you're one of the five percent. "Unlikely," the doctor will mumble while filling out an order for yet another test.

Here is an example. Sixty-six-year-old Hermione Barcrand (not her real name) went to a university general medical clinic to get something for a nagging bad cold. She happened to see a lung specialist who also spent one session a week in the general medicine clinic. A chest x-ray was ordered and there was a large and troublesome shadow on the x-ray in the middle of her chest, in the space between her lungs. She hadn't lost weight, her appetite was good, and, except for the bad cold that was hanging on, she felt fine. The doctor learned from Ms. Barcrand that she had had a chest x-ray a year earlier at the local health department as a screen for tuberculosis. The health department informed her that she did not have TB but that there was something abnormal on her x-ray that she should see someone about. She had not seen a doctor since then. The clinic doctor gave her some medicines for her cold and asked her to return to the clinic in two weeks.

When Ms. Barcrand returned two weeks later, her cold was gone and the doctor had good news for her. He had gotten hold of the health department x-ray done a year earlier and it showed exactly the same shadow that was there now. The shadow had not changed at all; if anything it was slightly smaller. The doctor had no idea what the shadow was, but since it had been there a long time, was causing Ms. Barcrand no difficulty, and hadn't changed, it was very unlikely to be anything to worry about. To find out for sure what the shadow was would have required several expensive, invasive, and risky tests. After discussion, the two of them agreed that she would return for repeat x-rays in six months and then probably annually if the shadow remained stable. A careful weighing of the available evidence with a sensible result that reassured the patient at limited cost was less risky for Ms. Barcrand than the tests that would have to be done to pin down a diagnosis. Medicine done the way it should be done.

But, there is more to the story. A year or so after the above described clinic visit, the doctor who was following Ms. Barcrand stopped working in the general clinic and she was assigned to a new primary care provider (PCP; we aren't sure when we stopped calling them doctors). This new PCP was apparently a committed disciple of the yes–or–no school of medicine. One look at the x-ray and Ms. Barcrand was told that she probably had cancer. CT scans of her chest and abdomen were done. They showed the mass in the middle of her chest but also a small shadow in her liver. "Aha!" the PCP no doubt thought. The cancer has spread from her chest to her liver. Plans were made to get a surgeon to open her chest and take a biopsy of the lesion. Ms. Barcrand, beside herself with the fear that she had a fatal cancer, contacted her original doctor, who organized a thorough review of her case by a panel of specialists. On a careful look, the radiologist decided that the shadow in her liver was probably a normal vein seen at an odd angle, and all agreed that if the mass in her chest was cancer it was unlike any cancer that any of them had ever seen. Ms. Barcrand was assured that although none of those specialists knew what resided in her chest, it almost certainly wasn't cancer. She had no further tests, but returned annually for a chest x-ray which remained completely unchanged for years. She narrowly escaped the avalanche of tests and other interventions that a doctor who had to have a definitive answer would have triggered.

But if you and this doctor get too deep into a problem, it may be difficult for either of you to see the situation with clear eyes. Neither of you may recognize that you have stepped onto a slippery slope that will cost a lot of money, put you at mortal risk, and will not make you healthier. And, unfortunately, there may not be a cooler head around to rescue you.

Michael Rothberg, a professor at the Cleveland Clinic, describes just such an experience of his aging father in an article in the *Journal of the American Medical Association* titled, "The $50,000 Physical." The story has been repeated elsewhere, but it is such an accurate real life illustration of the possible consequences of this yes-or-no approach to medicine that it bears another telling.

Dr. Rothberg's eighty-five-year-old father moved with his wife into an assisted living facility in a new locale. He had only a couple of minor health problems. Shortly after relocating, he went for a checkup with his new primary care provider. When the doctor palpated the gentleman's stomach he thought the aorta, the main artery in the abdomen, was too prominent and wondered whether there was an aneurysm, a swelling of the aorta that can be serious, even fatal. An ultrasound study showed a normal aorta, but something suspicious in the pancreas, so the doctor ordered a CT scan of the area. The CT scan showed a normal pancreas, but there was a worrisome shadow in the liver. The patient had an occupational history of exposure to organic chemicals over his many working years, and the doctor knew that exposure to these chemicals was sometimes associated with liver cancer. Mr. Rothberg felt fine. He was unaware of any problem with his liver. But his physician sent him to a specialist who felt that this thing in his liver had to be biopsied to find out if it was a cancer. So Mr. Rothberg was admitted to the hospital for the procedure which involves sticking a large needle through the abdominal wall into the liver and removing a small core of tissue. Well, it wasn't cancer. It was a localized tangle of blood vessels called a hemangioma and sticking a big needle into a tangle of blood vessels is not a good idea. Mr. Rothberg bled profusely into his abdomen, requiring transfusion of ten pints of blood. He was in a lot of pain and almost died. The total bill for all this was, as the title of the article says, $50,000. So the doctor's curiosity was satisfied, but at exorbitant cost in dollars and human suffering and with absolutely no benefit to Mr. Rothberg. This doctor, as someone said of a preacher after a too long Sunday sermon, missed a lot of good stopping places.

What would our good doctor have done differently? She certainly would have called a halt to the fiasco somewhere early in the course of things and sent Mr. Rothberg on his merry way with his wife to enjoy his new home for whatever time he had left. But how would the doctor have known when to quit? There is no clear and unambiguous answer to that; if there were, this man's doctor might have restrained himself. A doctor more comfortable with uncertainty would know that some people think that there is no reason to even do an exam on a person who has no complaints. She would also know that feeling the stomach of an elderly man is not likely to tell you much of anything specific. Then having felt something abnormal and done an ultrasound, should you chase after a shadow in the pancreas? Not clear. Cancers of the pancreas are devilishly hard to cure, but the best chance is if you find it early. So there was a maybe at every stage of this man's workup. Deciding what and what not to pursue means knowing the available evidence, but understanding it in the context of this specific person and circumstance. In fact, with exactly the same evidence in hand, the decision may differ in different people and different situations. A single well-timed *maybe* would have served this patient much better than a battery of noes and saved him or his insurance company $50K to boot. Choosing when and where to deploy the maybe requires knowledge, understanding, and a level of comfort with uncertainty.

The doctor hell-bent on a definitive answer to every question bears some responsibility for the high cost of health care. The dogged pursuit of a yes or no answer that may not be critical to your care can lead to excessive use of expensive tests. A coalition of medical societies has formed a *Choosing Wisely* project that has created lists of tests and treatments that most doctors agree are done too often. Some examples are exercise tests for heart disease in people without symptoms who are not at high risk, extensive imaging tests for low back pain, CT scans and MRIs for headaches, and bone density scans in women at low risk for osteoporosis. In each case, not only are the tests expensive, but they are likely to precipitate more tests, magnifying expenses without improving care. In 2009, just twelve medical tests deemed by expert review to have been done without an adequate indication cost the system $6.8 billion. The human cost is unknown but chances are it is really big.

A doctor who is determined to get an answer can call on a frightening array of technologies and there are few restraints. *"Nobody ever gets sued for ordering unnecessary tests,"* says Arizona generalist Doug Campos-Outcalt. The lure of ever proliferating technology to one not comfortable with ambiguity is irresistible. Some choose the profession primarily because they fall head over heels in love with the technology and, as often happens in passionate love affairs, they can lose their perspective. Technology, in perspective, is a fabulous addition to medicine, but best to avoid doctors too much enthralled by it. They really are in the wrong business.

Given all that, how does this doctor stay in business? Why don't his patients see that the doctor rather than the patient is at the center of this relationship and move on? At some point shouldn't it become clear that you are paying a lot of money and taking unnecessary risks primarily to satisfy the doctor's need for certainty?

There are probably several reasons for doctors to take this yes-or-no approach, but an important one is that we all want certain answers to questions about our health; it's a human tendency. In fact, a compelling reason to avoid this kind of doctor is that you are a human being and therefore a set-up for a *folie à deux*, a relationship that exploits your own discomfort with uncertainty and loses the focus on making your health as good as it can be. You have to rely on your doctor to help you understand that the best answer can be *maybe*, a foreign concept to the doctor with a yes-or-no obsession.

The human tendency to want an unequivocal answer even without a clear question is illustrated in a study of men's reactions to measurements of the level of prostate specific antigen (PSA) in their blood. Although there is controversy in this area, there is some evidence that a markedly elevated PSA suggests the possibility of prostate cancer. The next level of test is a biopsy of the prostate gland. That is not a very complicated procedure, but it is invasive, uncomfortable, and with some risk. In this study forty percent of men whose PSA measurement was equivocal, that is, "provides no information about whether or not you have cancer," when given the choice, still opted for going ahead with a biopsy. Even when there is nothing to explain about the test results, no information one way or the other, not even a maybe, we still want to exhaust every remote possibility. Most of us are prime candidates for this doctor's brand of black or white medicine.

The doctor who has trouble dealing with uncertainty is stuck with a concept of diagnosis as a dichotomy, like a true/false test. But human disease is not a short answer quiz. It is a very private essay. Your doctor's job is to understand your unique health-disease narrative and use that to help decide what questions to ask and, from among the extensive menu of possible tests, which ones are likely to give information that will make a difference. This breed of doctor doesn't ask questions if getting at the answers involves subjecting you to risk, expense, discomfort, or inconvenience unless the answers are likely to cause a change in your care, no matter how interesting she might find the answers. There is a place for research in human beings and we hope that you will volunteer for such studies if you're asked to, but that brand of research must be done with full disclosure, according to strict rules, and with objective and diligent oversight. Your health care is not about satisfying the intellectual curiosity of your doctor, it's about doing what is best for you.

But how can you know whether the tests your doctor orders are reasonable, appropriate, and necessary for your optimal health care or whether they're being ordered primarily to satisfy the doctor's desire to know the answer? There are some clues and also some things you can do to flush out this doctor's real motives.

Does your doctor explain the reason for tests, the risks involved, and how the results will or will not affect your care? If not, you should ask those questions, but if it comes to that, you might start to wonder whether you and the doctor are on the same page. You are supposed to be the focus of this relationship and it is hard to believe that to be true if you're not told what's going on. The doctor who is laser focused on getting a definitive answer to every question is often not long on explaining her actions; she really doesn't see the point. She's determined to get the answers and you just happen to be her current source material.

You should *never hesitate to get another opinion* of the plan for diagnosing your condition and recommendations for what to do about it. This is especially true if things get complicated and expensive and invasive tests are in the offing, therapies with serious possible side effects are suggested, or there is a series of interventions that are progressively more risky (beware the slippery slope). Insisting on another professional opinion may well not please this doctor. In fact if she is too displeased with or threatened by such a request, that's a pretty reliable clue that you may not have chosen the best health care collaborator. You should never be intimidated by the displeasure of your doctor. You're not there to make her happy. You're there because you need the doctor's help and if the two of you can't work together on your problem amiably, the result is not likely to be as good as it ought to be.

If there is anything that you don't understand or are unsure about, you should *ask as many questions as needed* to be sure that you've got it right. That isn't likely to make this doc happy, but that's her problem. You should just keep asking the questions until you're satisfied. Sincere questions politely asked will not annoy the good doctor; she will answer them in kind.

The questions you need to ask will depend on your personal needs, how much information your doctor volunteers, and the specific health related situation. But you need to be totally honest about what you need to know. The U.S. government's Agency for Health Care Research and Quality suggests the following ten questions to consider as a starting point. It is clear from this list that you need not be shy about being specific:

1. What is the test for?
2. How many times have you done this procedure?
3. When will I get the results?
4. Why do I need this treatment?
5. Are there any alternatives?
6. What are the possible complications?
7. Which hospital is best for my needs?
8. How do you spell the name of that drug?
9. Are there any side effects?
10. Will this medicine interact with medicines that I'm already taking?

Questions like these will go a long way toward revealing this doctor's true colors. Best to get that done early. If this relationship isn't going to work for you, the sooner you realize that and move on, the healthier you will be.

With the obsessive yes–or–no brand of medicine you will pay too much for care that is not as good as it should be and sometimes carries unnecessary risks. The same is true of a doctor who believes that she knows all the answers—we're about to meet one of those in the next chapter.

CHAPTER 6

The Infallibility Illusion

What the good doctor doesn't know could save your life and what this doctor "knows" could do you some serious harm. That almost happened to Susan Black (not her real name). It would have, too, if she hadn't taken matters into her own hands. We can learn something important from Susan Black.

When Ms. Black discovered a golf ball size lump on her chest, she immediately consulted her family doctor. She had no pain, she hadn't lost any weight, and she felt perfectly fine. The lump just appeared out of the blue. She was referred to a surgeon who removed the lump and finally, after waiting two agonizing weeks, she was told that two pathologists had reviewed the biopsy and concluded that it was a "panniculitis-like T-cell lymphoma," a rare cancer that could very well kill her and that required immediate treatment. She was referred to an oncologist who ordered extensive blood tests and a CT scan. When she protested to the oncologist that she felt fine he responded that the periodic hot flashes she was having were symptoms from her tumor. "But," she said, "I'm fifty-two! At fifty-two all women have night sweats and hot flashes." She asked whether there wasn't a chance that the lab results were wrong, and he replied absolutely not and encouraged her not to delay starting treatment. When she told him that she wanted a second opinion before con-senting to start his recommended chemotherapy, the doctor responded, "What you have is so rare, no one will know any more about it than I do." Fortunately, Ms. Black, no fan of the myth of the infallible doctor, didn't buy that. She did consult another expert, who reviewed all of her test data including the biopsy and concluded that she didn't have cancer at all, but rather a completely benign lesion that would resolve without treatment. She had no therapy and continued in good health, narrowly escaping certain misery from the oncologist's supremely confident recommendations.

What Ms. Black's doctor knew for certain, like many medical certainties, turned out to be wrong. All of the doctors involved here, the internist, the pathologist, and the oncologist, were too sure of themselves and the attitude of each reinforced certainty in the others. Ms. Black was in danger of being caught up in a positive feedback loop resonating among her multiple doctors that was leading her full tilt in the wrong direction. Although the root cause of that situation may have included arrogance, we suspect knowledge without understanding was the real problem. The pathologist said it was cancer so the internist referred her to a cancer doctor and the cancer doctor did what he was trained to do, choose a chemo regimen based on the pathologist's diagnosis and move on. But they were all wrong because nobody paused to consider the possibility that there was something worrisome about this case. Fortunately Ms. Black found a doctor who was more open to alternative explanations for her problem, but she had to summon the courage to challenge the confident recommendations of several experts to get there. And it took her four tries!

You should not confuse your doctor's confidence in her

expertise with how right she is about your condition. In fact, how certainly the overconfident doctor answers your questions may have nothing to do with whether or not she's right. British pediatric neurosurgeon Richard Hayward observes of doctors' attitudes, "Infallibility refutes the possibility of error to which all human beings are susceptible. Authority is the uniform it wears." You can be absolutely certain that your doctor is not infallible. If she mistakes her white coat for a uniform of authority, you should take your business elsewhere.

Knowledge, whether a little or a lot, is dangerous. History is full of examples. Knowledge implies certainty and certainty has done a lot of mischief—driven religious intolerance, perpetuated scientific error, distorted our understanding of cosmology, and caused doctors to harm the very people they were sworn to help. The idea that doctors have irrefutable knowledge may have its roots in an era when shaman healers laid claim to a spiritual inside track. Shedding the claim of a special connection to God may be progress, but there are still too many doctors around who relish their roles as unquestionable authorities. It doesn't serve their charges well. The doctor who knows all the answers doesn't understand the information; uncertainty is hard wired to understanding. The all-knowing doctor is lying to herself and the doctor who lies to herself will, inevitably, deceive her patients.

As happened with Ms. Black, the doctor who's too certain can hurt you by missing the diagnosis and so prescribing the wrong therapy. She can also be so certain that she knows all of the possible effective therapies that she keeps you from getting something innovative that might save your life.

Although hopefully this happens rarely, it does happen and the results can be tragic.

Here is a deeply painful tragedy, the blame for which lies squarely at the feet of an overconfident doctor. A man getting chemotherapy in his small local hospital was responding well without complications. His cancer was improving and it looked like he would recover. After a regular treatment late on a Friday, he developed diarrhea. By the next day the diarrhea was so severe that his wife took him to the local emergency room. He was admitted to the hospital and found to have an infection of his bowels with the dangerous bacterium, *Clostridium difficile* (*C. diff*). That is not a rare complication of chemotherapy, but it is a serious one that is devilishly difficult to treat and can be fatal. The patient got rapidly worse until he was nearing death in spite of antibiotics. His wife had a friend who had had chronic *C. diff* diarrhea that did not respond to antibiotics but was essentially cured by a fecal transplant. From the internet, they learned that this still experimental treatment could cure resistant *C. diff* diarrhea in up to ninety percent of cases. The patient's wife pleaded with the doctor to try it. Her husband was nearing death and nothing seemed to be working. What was there to lose? The doctor said that he had never heard of fecal transplant therapy. When she continued to plead with him to reconsider, the doctor refused to discuss it further, telling her that he didn't want to hear any more of her "bullshit quackery." The next day, the patient died. He died for want of a doctor with the knowledge, understanding, courage, and human decency to entertain the possibility that maybe there was something he did not know.

And this attitude of infallibility can develop early. A

nurse in a Washington hospital was alarmed when she saw that her patient who had a shunt in place to drain fluid from his brain was vomiting and complaining of headache. She knew those were symptoms of increasing pressure in his brain, probably because the shunt had clotted off and stopped draining the fluid. When she called the resident on duty who was sleeping in the hospital, he told her not to worry about it. But she did worry about it, a lot. After a while when the patient's symptoms didn't improve, she called the resident a second time to which he responded, "You don't know what to look for—you're not a doctor!" and slammed down the phone. Fortunately for the patient, the nurse called the attending doctor and the patient was treated appropriately, narrowly escaping serious brain injury or death. We don't know whatever happened to the resident; surely he was severely chastised for this kind of behavior. We hope he learned from that experience, but we fear that he may be practicing medicine somewhere, supremely confident of his exceptional knowledge and thoroughly certain that he rarely if ever makes mistakes.

But that resident still makes mistakes, no matter how much he knows. It's said that preventable medical mistakes account for a sixth of all annual deaths in the U.S., and we'd bet a lot that overconfident doctors account for more than their fair share of those errors.

So you don't want the services of an overconfident doctor because she makes too many mistakes. She does that in many ways—by doing the wrong thing, by assuming she knows something that she doesn't, and by failing to look beyond her headlights. Here is an example of a doctor who was so confident of the diagnosis that he didn't look for anything beyond his immediate field of vision. After all, he knew what was wrong with the patient. Why look any further?

A Washington pediatrician had practiced medicine for forty years when his throat started hurting. He arranged to see a doctor about it and after recounting his symptoms he was told that his throat pain was due to reflux of acid from his stomach backing up into his esophagus. He went home and did as he was told but the pain didn't go away. He revisited the doctor and was told again that his problem was acid reflux. Finally, after seven months of this, the patient happened to see an astute resident who decided to look down his throat using a simple technique commonly done by ENT doctors. Lo and behold, there sat a cancer, "the size of a peach pit." The cancer was cured by completely removing the patient's voice box, but what if the doctor he saw at first hadn't been so sure of himself and had taken a look seven months earlier? An arrogant doctor doesn't know what he doesn't know.

What happens behind the scenes can also impact your care, even though you rarely get a good look at the back office operations. An arrogant doctor doesn't always behave well back there. When cornered, this doc can turn mean and the consequences aren't good. In one survey, 67 percent of health care workers at 102 nonprofit hospitals believed that doctors' disruptive behavior caused medical mistakes, and eighteen percent reported firsthand knowledge of a medical mistake caused by an obnoxious doctor.

Highly opinionated and defensive doctors also cause collateral damage by creating an unpleasant and threatening environment that makes it difficult for other health professionals to do a good job. The stress of the operating room can bring out a surgeon's worst—thrown scalpels, demeaning epithets hurled at assistants, irrational outbursts of temper. It happens on medical wards too. An attending doctor flings a patient's chart clear across a nurses' station at a cowering intern who failed to get a requested test done on time (that actually happened more than once in an elite medical institution). A survey by the *Institute for Safe Medication Practices* says that forty percent of hospital staff report being so intimidated by a doctor that they dared not raise questions about apparently incorrect medicine orders. The arrogant doctor leaves casualties—colleagues and patients—in her wake. You don't want to be one of them.

And heaven help us if the "infallible" doctor winds up in charge of writing guidelines that are imposed on the other doctors practicing in his system. Guidelines can be misunderstood as implying unyielding certainty, and wind up being used to coerce doctors into uniform application of a practice. This kind of thing plays right into the overconfident doctor's hands. The problem is that there are always *maybes*, exceptions to virtually any guideline that anyone can write. So you may stand to benefit from a rigid application of a guideline that benefits most people. Or you may not.

For example, there are guidelines that recommend giving a heart drug called a beta blocker (how it works is not important to the point) to patients getting anesthesia for a heart operation. At least in some cases, insurance companies require that this be done in a very high percent (preferably 100) of patients in this category or they won't pay. So, institutions go to great lengths to get anesthesiologists to give the drug—computer popup reminders, admonishments from administrators, constant review of the success rate, etc. With the imprimatur of the power structure behind the practice, the doctor can be absolutely certain of what do to; don't think about it, just give the drug. The overconfident doctor loves this stuff. However, there are some patients who are likely to be harmed rather than helped by a beta blocker. If a doctor is caring for a patient whom he is pretty sure is in that category, what does he do? Powerful organizational and financial forces say give the drug anyway, while that pesky dictum of Hippocrates to which a doctor is sworn—*primum non nocere*—says safety of the patient is paramount. There was a memo from the chief of anesthesia congratulating the group on 100 percent compliance with the practice over the past several months and warning that missing giving the drug to even one patient would drop the group out of the top 10 percent of peer institutions and risk decreased payments from the insurance company—damned if you do, damned if you don't.

No problem, says the supremely confident doctor. If she fears that the patient is likely to be harmed by the drug, she should give a very small dose (sub-therapeutic is the medical term) of a very short acting form of beta blocker. Then everyone is happy. The box in the patient's record that says a beta blocker was given can be truthfully checked, but the patient is spared any effect of the drug. The result? Consistently 99 percent compliance; everybody's happy. This is the kind of ludicrous practice that certainty of universal benefit can cause. What's best for you is not front and center in this situation. Front and center is getting a check mark in the box that will assure compliance with a universal guideline. But no universal guideline is really universal. If your doctor tells you anything is 100 percent effective, don't believe it!

But perhaps we're being too hard on the self-confident doctor. There is a place for *informed* certainty in medicine. In fact there are situations in which a doctor needs to have the courage and confidence to act on the best available information. In some circumstances, the right thing for you is for the doctor to do something . . . now. Your life could depend on it. You don't want a timid surgeon!

A middle-aged professional acquaintance of ours needed an operation to remove a cancerous tumor. A friend asked him, "How do you like the guy who's going to be cutting you open?" The man replied, "I feel the same way about the surgeon as I do about the pilot who flies an airplane that I'm on. Whether or not I like her is irrelevant. What is relevant is that she knows what she's doing and does it really well." Doctors, especially surgeons, must be decisive at times and they have to be convinced that what they are doing is the right thing or they won't do it well. And you won't do as well unless you believe that your doctor makes good decisions and is skilled at her job.

One of us was once described by a Yale professor as being "unencumbered by knowledge." While we are quite sure that the Yale professor didn't intend that as a compliment, there is a sense in which knowledge can get in the way of understanding; the Canadian environmentalist, Farley Mowat, admonishes, "never let the facts get in the way of truth." And it's not only, as Alexander Pope says in his famous poem, a little learning that is dangerous. We fear that those in medicine who drink most deeply of Pope's Pierian spring are sometimes the scariest. That's because there can be a false sense of certainty that comes from memorizing what for the time being pass for answers, forgetting how ephemeral answers can be—losing one's sense of *maybe*. On occasion, knowledge can close the mind to new possibilities. That is no excuse for failing to learn from the available information; you don't want a dumb doctor. But you don't want a doctor who doesn't know when he is wrong either. If we pay attention we can learn by being wrong.

So how can you avoid getting involved with a know-it-all doctor and realizing it too late, after something goes seriously awry? Here are some things to look out for:

- *This doctor is not at all interested in partnering; she is completely in charge and has no patience with any challenge to her authority.* She pays little attention to what you have to say. She might respond to your question with, "I am the doctor here, don't tell me how to do my job!" Or she might say, "Just do what I tell you to. There's a reason we call them doctor's orders."

- *The doctor is disrespectful to staff and/or other health care professionals.* Although this doctor's worst behavior will likely happen elsewhere, there may be clues in how she talks to nurses, aids, and other personnel while tending to you. How members of her staff behave in her presence can also betray less than amiable relationships. Are they overly deferential? Do they appear frightened of the doctor? One of the staff may make an apparently off-handed comment when the doctor's not around about how difficult she is to work with; that's a red flag.

○ *The doctor appears sleepy or seems to have trouble concentrating.* Sleep deprivation can cause even the most well-intentioned doctor to be impatient and short tempered, to act like a jerk. Doctors may be more likely than most people to have their sleep interrupted by the demands of a busy practice, and paradoxically, they may not realize how seriously chronic loss of sleep is changing their behavior for the worse. A tactful observation that your doctor seems tired might call her attention to the problem and could even help to change her behavior. However, if the problem persists, you will just have to admit that this person may be incorrigibly arrogant whether or not she is sleep derived.

○ *The doctor is disrespectful to other patients.* While you shouldn't deliberately eavesdrop, sometimes you may hear the doctor talking to another patient or discussing a patient on the telephone. If that happens, *pay attention to how the patient is addressed or referred to.* The know-it-all doctor doesn't always show appropriate respect for her patients even when they are face to face and commits even worse offenses when discussing a case with a colleague.

Reflecting on a visit to the doctor, do you feel that:

- **O**   You were dealt with as a mature and reasonably intelligent adult?

- **O**   Your problem was the central issue?

- **O**   The doctor adequately explained what she thought was wrong and how she planned to proceed?

- **O**   You and the doctor talked to, not at, each other?

Remember, you choose your doctor, not the other way around. While your choices may be limited, you do not have to accept poor treatment—at least not without exploring all of the available possibilities. You should make every effort to create a good working partnership, as discussed earlier, but if the relationship still isn't working you should do your best to find a better situation.

We can only hope that the next candidate in line is not the chronically unhappy person whom we are about to meet in the next chapter.

CHAPTER 7

The "Poor Me" Syndrome

You don't want a doctor who is unhappy with the job and the odds that you may wind up with one appear to be increasing. Perhaps you can understand the situation better by looking at the size of the problem, some reasons for it, and some of the potential consequences. While understanding the situation may not overwhelm you with sympathy for the doctor suffering from this "poor me" malady, it might help you to avoid some real health risks on your way to finding a doctor who better appreciates uncertainty.

Most doctors claim that they chose their career for noble reasons, although definitions of nobility vary. The claim to care for one's fellow humans is pretty common, but expectations of a higher than average income, prominent social status, general respect, and admiration of family and peers are also pretty high on many doctors' lists of reasons for choosing a medical career.

Whatever their expectations were when they started out, a lot of doctors no longer like their job. There is a catalogue of complaints—overwork, underpay, lack of respect, fear of lawsuits, pressure to over-test, bloated schedules, cumbersome electronic medical records, etc. In a survey of twelve thousand physicians only six percent described their morale as positive. Sandeep Juahar, author of *Doctored*, says, "American doctors are suffering from a collective malaise. We strove, made sacrifices—and for what? For many of us the job has become only that—a job."

Many doctors feel that they are victims of a failing system, forced to compromise their practice standards, and pressured into a profit driven style of health care that they do not enjoy and is different than what they expected. Those feelings are proliferating; there are more and more unhappy doctors. Fifty-eight percent of two thousand physicians surveyed several years ago said their enthusiasm for medicine had been on the wane for five years; eighty-seven percent said their morale was sinking. Over one eight-year period the number of doctors who doubted that they were in the right profession increased from around ten percent to nearly half. A lot of a thousand-plus doctors questioned in 2009 said they had moderate to severe problems with feelings of isolation, work-life stress, or dissatisfaction. The long list of reasons given for disintegrating doctor job satisfaction is readily condensed to just two—time and money.

There are two parts to the time problem—too little of it and too little control of how it's spent. Doctors complain that the excessive commercialization of health care has turned their lives over to managers. Doctors are *providers*, a *resource* to be *optimally deployed* to *maximize efficiency*. Terms and phrases like those are relatively recent additions to the health care conversation. Demands to get more patients through the system faster have dramatically shrunk the amount of time a doctor actually spends with a patient. Couple that with the time spent documenting virtually everything, contracting with a variety of payers, and desperately trying to establish a meaningful relationship with a clunky electronic medical record, and one might start to feel like a lot of physicians who said to Jay Crosson, vice president of professional satisfaction for the American Medical Association, "I used to be a doctor, now I'm a clerk."

When doctors are asked what about their practice other than money gives them the greatest feeling of satisfaction, most answer things like, "relationships with my patients," "making a difference in peoples' lives," "providing good medical care." But those things take time, and there is a pervasive notion that the basic principle driving medical practice is, "time is money" and so a commodity that must be doled out with careful attention to the economics. It's not surprising that around half of 7,200 doctors surveyed by the Mayo Clinic in 2012 reported at least one symptom of burnout (formally defined as a combination of emotional exhaustion, feelings of depersonalization, and decreased sense of personal accomplishment).

What are these thieves of time that rob doctors of the satisfaction they expected from their profession? As we said above, one is the demand to see more patients faster; half of practicing primary care physicians spend less than sixteen minutes with each patient they see. Many think that number is shrinking. Some visits don't require much time, especially for a patient whom the doctor knows well. But establishing that critical relationship starts with a thorough history and physical examination. It's not obvious what kind of a history and physical examination can be done in less than sixteen minutes, but it is virtually certain that such an effort would not have met with Professor Osler's approval. Stanford physician and author Abraham Verghese makes the point most elegantly in his TED talk "A Doctor's Touch." The process of taking a history and doing a physical exam is about more than getting information. It is an essential part of creating that "relationship with a patient" that doctors claim is a main source of their job satisfaction. And it takes time!

Then there is the eternally proliferating "paperwork," the requirements for highly specific and complete documentation of absolutely everything that a doctor does or thinks. That, too, takes time. Two-thirds of primary care providers spend ten hours or more each week doing paperwork and administration. One could do at least ten Oslerian-level patient histories and physical exams in ten hours. The electronic medical record and other wonders of the information age that promised doctors freedom from the burden of paperwork have turned out to eat up even more time. There are many reasons for that and, in the long run, electronics will make doctors more efficient, but the growing pains are excruciating.

The "poor me" doctor also believes that she is being underpaid and strongly suspects that the lion's share of the patient care dollars that she generates goes to administrators, managers, and other business types. All but five percent of the explosive growth in the health care workforce in recent years has been more administrators, not more doctors. That may be one reason why half of practicing doctors do not feel "fairly compensated" for what they do. They think that they are being ripped off by the suits. In fact, some believe that the serious time problem driving doctors to burnout is at root a money problem. Has medical practice metamorphosed from a caring activity with doctors' relationships with patients as a core value into an essentially commercial enterprise managed by generously compensated *suits* and driven more by the health of the bottom line than the health of the people responsible for paying the bill?

Some people think that's true (other books have been written on the subject), but let's focus on doctors' incomes. Are the half of practicing doctors who feel underpaid all suffering from the "poor me" syndrome? Well, there are almost certainly doctors who are not fairly compensated for what they do, and some fraction of those who believe that to be true no doubt have a case. But consider some facts. In 2015, the average annual salary of a primary care doctor was $195,000; for specialties the number was $284,000. Incomes exclusively from patient care ranged from $189,000 for pediatricians to $421,000 for orthopedic surgeons. Data from 2009 indicate that cumulative lifetime earnings were about $6.5 million for primary care doctors and more than $10 million for specialists. Granted, doctors spend many years and many dollars (often borrowed dollars that must be repaid) getting educated and trained, and there are plenty of people in our country who invested a lot less time and money preparing for their job and yet make a lot more money than doctors. Sandeep Jauhar, quoted earlier, points out in *Doctored* that people who choose medicine have a lot of other career options where they could make more money and there is some truth to that. However, median household annual income in the U.S. is currently about $50,000. That means that there are plenty of people whose income is less than that. And unpaid medical bills are the leading cause of this year's two million bankruptcies. You will probably have trouble feeling a lot of sympathy for a doctor complaining about a $200K salary, not to mention for the half million dollar a year orthopedist. We agree with Dr. Jauhar that if minimizing educational requirements and maximizing income are very high on one's list of criteria for choosing a profession one should probably look somewhere other than medicine. But doctors are assured plenty of income to support a very good life regardless of their areas of practice; they live better than most of their fellow countrymen. You should be wary of the doctor who complains too loudly about the salary that goes with the job.

There are a lot of reasons why you don't need to feel too bad for the doctor who doesn't like her job, no matter how miserable she sounds. For one thing, a secure and well-paying job these days is not to be taken lightly. And, after all, doctors are not indentured servants. Medical skills are marketable and there are still many professional options in this country. If a doctor feels that her practice is demeaning, insensitive, and over-demanding, perhaps she should consider looking for another job.

Martin Karnovsky and Janis Finer both did that. Dr. Karnovsky, a sixty-one-year-old internist in Chevy Chase, Maryland, was seeing patients every fifteen minutes. He hated it. He worried that he was missing important things and knew that he was short-changing the people he was trying to care for. He worked with a consultant who helps doctors switch to a concierge model and reduced his patient load from 1,200 to four hundred who pay more for longer visits and twenty-four-hour access to him; both he and his patients are happier. Dr. Finer, a fifty-seven-year-old primary care doctor in Tulsa left a busy practice for full time work in a hospital (she became a specialist known as a hospitalist) with predictable hours, every other week off, and increased pay—more time, more money. There are many such examples. Doctors have skills and knowledge that are valuable in the marketplace and they can take control of their professional lives if they choose to.

There are some other, perhaps more unusual options. If a doctor who is unhappy with the profession really wanted a job where she could take the time to practice medicine that connected with people and favorably affected her life, she could check with Dr. Victoria Sweet at the Laguna Honda hospital in San Francisco. *Slow medicine*, Dr. Sweet called it in her memoir, *God's Hotel*. Dr. Sweet took as much time as she needed to care for the penniless drug addicts, schizophrenics, and ailing elderly at Laguna Honda. And it worked for both Dr. Sweet and her patients. She felt good about her job and she saw things other doctors had missed.

For example, there was an elderly patient who had had recent hip surgery and who was diagnosed with Alzheimer's disease at another hospital. She was given antipsychotic drugs and taken from her home and her mentally disabled daughter. Dr. Sweet took some time with the patient and realized that the problem was not mental deterioration, it was pain from her replaced hip slipping out of its socket. Serious pain can occupy so much of one's brain that normal functions don't work as well. But it takes time for a doctor to discover that.

So a position at a place like Laguna Honda might be good therapy for the "poor me" syndrome. It could solve the time problem. The salary might not meet expectations, but it would be plenty to live on well enough and, hey, nobody ever promised Utopia. If more doctors tried *slow medicine* they might discover something good about themselves and their profession and all of us might benefit.

There are several practical reasons why you don't want any of the chronic complainers for your personal doctor if you can avoid it. For one thing, visits to such a doctor will not make you happy and that matters to your health. Both your attitude and that of your doctor affect the outcomes of your interactions for better or for worse. Danielle Ofri, author of *What Doctors Feel: How Emotions Affect the Practice of Medicine*, says that patients of high empathy doctors have 40 percent fewer severe complications of their diabetes than patients of low empathy doctors. Forty percent! That's as good as you can do with intensive medical therapy. So, you would do well to avoid an unhappy doctor because that relationship will make you unhappy and your health will suffer as a result.

Unhappy doctors also make more than their share of mistakes. The last thing you need is a consequence of a medical error, and avoiding that is hard enough even with a happy doctor. Somewhere between fifty thousand and two hundred thousand people die each year in American hospitals of preventable medical errors; patient harm has been said to be the third most frequent cause of death in the nation. Those errors are not committed by institutions; they are committed by people. Some of those people are doctors and it is very likely that many of the guilty parties are prone to being distracted by worries about the things that are wrong with their job; distracted doctors make mistakes.

In one study of seven hundred surgeons who believed they had made a medical error in the past three months, over two-thirds thought their errors were caused by burnout. The numbers of medical errors have prompted some alarmists to opine that conventional medicine "kills more people than it saves." That isn't true. There are too many medical mistakes, any is too many, but that opinion ignores the noble and effective efforts of the many dedicated, knowledgeable, and empathetic doctors of the world. While the fact that there are too many medical mistakes is not a fair indictment of the entire system, it does mean that you need to pay careful attention when selecting the people and places involved in your health care. It almost certainly means that you should avoid doctors suffering from the "poor me" syndrome.

Are doctors hapless victims of a diabolical health care system or can they do something to improve their lot? There probably is not a simple answer to that question, but there is a basic principle that the "poor me" syndrome may obscure. The critical people in any health care system are the health professionals—doctors, nurses, and others—and the patients, but the culture is largely driven by managers and other business types. The managers of the health care business need doctors and patients to manage or they have no business. If enough doctors refused to enable a viciously profit-driven practice that they claim to hate and enough patients refused to patronize such practices (patients are also dissatisfied with them), then the culture might be forced to change. More doctors would necessarily grow into open-minded and caring professionals who were comfortable with uncertainty or they'd be out of business.

So as you go about trying to locate for yourself that kind of doctor, you should keep a keen eye out for symptoms of the "poor me" syndrome. Although doctor "burn-out" is a serious and increasing problem that needs to be addressed by the profession, your relationship with your doctor should be focused on *your* health. It will only depress you to be subjected to a litany of travails of the profession, and that will not make you healthier.

PART III

Some Things That Your Doctor Should Know

. . . And Why They Matter

CHAPTER 8

The Difference between "Facts" and Facts

There is nothing more deceptive than an obvious fact.
—ARTHUR CONAN DOYLE, "The Boscombe Valley Mystery"

The good doctor is very suspicious of things that *everybody knows*. There are too many examples of accepted "facts" based on popular beliefs that turn out not to be true. For example, everybody knows that Sherlock Holmes was fond of responding to a compliment of his deductive powers from his colleague with the words, "Elementary, my dear Watson." But what everybody knows in that case is not true. The great detective spoke all of those words on multiple occasions, but did not once speak them linked together. One could call that the "everybody knows fallacy." There is a long list of *obvious facts*, things everybody knows, that are untrue; conventional wisdom may be conventional, but it is not reliably wise.

The good doctor also knows that a lot of harm can come from believing "facts" loudly proclaimed by public figures whose opinions are at odds with the best science and even by so-called experts whose judgment is clouded by a personal agenda—the "celebrity expert fallacy."

Here is an example. British gastroenterologist Andrew Wakefield and colleagues published a paper in 1998 claiming that vaccinating children against infectious diseases caused autism. The paper was subsequently retracted by the journal and there is no credible evidence that supports the claim. However, that paper has become "the holy text" of the anti-vaccine movement. That movement, energized by various celebrities with wide exposure as well as by Dr. Wakefield's efforts in the popular media, almost certainly shares responsibility for the failure of a number of children to get the MMR [measles, mumps, rubella (German measles)] triple vaccine. That vaccine is one of the most dramatic success stories in the history of childhood medicine. More unvaccinated children in the population risks an epidemic and fatalities.

This is not just a theoretical risk. Although measles was eliminated from the U.S. a couple of decades ago, that doesn't mean that in this decade your unvaccinated child is safe from a disease with potential complications of encephalitis, pneumonia, and even death. Measles and other childhood infections are still common in large parts of the world. So the parents of a kid from one of those places take their child on her dream trip to Disneyland, unaware that she is incubating the measles virus. In Anaheim the kid, infectious but not yet sick, bumps into unvaccinated children from all over America as the happy family ambles about the theme park. Then the kid comes down with a full blown case of measles and is the index case for a large multi-state measles outbreak. We didn't make this up. Something like this actually happened in 2015. And in 2019, a similar situation occurred in New York.

This good doctor knows that withholding vaccination puts children at risk for a variety of preventable diseases and invites recurrence of epidemics of infectious diseases that have all but disappeared. She also knows that *most medical opinions of celebrities are worse than useless as evidence.* She'll help you make sure that you're not dazzled into making bad health decisions by either glib hucksters or the seductive glamour of celebrities. As just one example, she will do everything in her power to see that you vaccinate your kids. This doctor has serious doubts about anything that everybody knows and has a healthy suspicion of facts, obvious or not, because she knows a thing or two about the nature of medical evidence.

Evidence-based medicine aims to rescue medical practice from the maw of myth, folklore, misguided opinion, and conventional wisdom and bring some rigor and consistency to the field. Hard to argue with the motive, but how do you and your doctor know what evidence to trust? How do we parse "facts" from facts?

In medicine as in the rest of life, questions have three possible answers—yes, no, or maybe; the drug (or operation or whatever) works, doesn't work, or there's not enough evidence to tell either way. Or there may be no rigorously analyzed data, no evidence at all. The old saw "absence of evidence is not evidence of absence" is true enough in medicine to give the good doctor pause before she becomes too dogmatic about anything. Nassim Nicholas Taleb's fascinating book, *The Black Swan*, referred to earlier, deals with this idea. A single black swan belied the prevailing concept that all swans were white. And you can never know whether there is an undiscovered exception lurking out there somewhere (one of Donald Rumsfeld's *unknown unknowns*) that will stand your solid reliable fact on its ear.

Well aware that not all "evidence" is created equal, the good doctor is a tenacious critic of medical dogma. She pays a lot of attention to where information comes from. One of her most valued sources is the Cochrane Collaboration.

When the Scottish doctor, Archibald Cochrane, was a captive of the Germans and caring for the unfortunate prisoners in World War II concentration camps, he became acutely aware of how precious little evidence there was to support most of what doctors did. Less speculation and folklore and more sound science is what he thought was needed to make the best conclusions about what did and didn't work. Cochrane's preoccupation with the need for carefully designed and controlled studies in people became his lifelong *raison d'être*. His 1971 book, *Effectiveness and Efficiency: Random Reflections on Health Services,* made an eloquent case for randomized controlled clinical trials, and Cochrane's effective advocacy for such trials eventually led to the international collaboration that bears his name. The Cochrane Collaboration is widely accepted as the premier source for critical evaluations of medical practices.

Given its origins, it is no surprise that the Cochrane Collaboration considers randomized controlled trials the best possible evidence, the gold standard, and most people agree that such studies (commonly abbreviated RCT) are the ideal. In such trials, groups of people with a given condition are treated with test intervention or a placebo. Who gets which is entirely random and the doctor doing the study doesn't know which patients get which treatment (the design is called "double blind," i.e., neither the patient nor the doctor knows what the treatment is). How many people are going to be studied is decided in advance and (barring something unforeseen) studies must be completed on that number of patients before the master code showing who got what is broken and the statisticians analyze the results. That's about as good as one can design a study to keep everybody honest and eliminate even unconscious bias on the part of the doctors involved.

The highest level of evidence, then, is the systematic evaluation of all of the relevant randomized controlled trials (assuming there are several and the more the better) in an area with a stated degree of certainty (statistical precision) of the conclusion. Cochrane's panels of experts scrutinize study designs for the potential for bias. They look at the size of any effect, whether what looks good to the statisticians is big enough to make any difference in the real world; statistical significance doesn't necessarily mean biologic significance. And then there's the source of funding for a study. There are, unfortunately, examples where a funding source with a dog in the fight could have unduly influenced what got into the published literature. There is no place for blind trust even in randomized controlled trials.

Cochrane reviews are daily fare for the good doctor. But she also read a 2010 *Atlantic* article titled "Lies, Damned Lies and Medical Science" that made her look a little more carefully at the work of statistician John Ioannidis, director of the Stanford Prevention Research Center. The article says that Ioannidis "and his team have shown, again and again, and in many different ways, that much of what biomedical researchers conclude in published studies . . . is misleading, exaggerated, and often flat-out wrong." Ioannidis opines that

90 percent of the published medical information that doctors use to decide how to treat their patients may be flawed. Dr. Ioannidis doesn't buy the RCT thing, at least not the way such studies are generally done.

Dr. Ioannidis says that conclusions of random controlled trials may be wrong because they are too small, too sensitive to small effects, too unselective (i.e., too many things are measured), too imprecise in design, or too dependent on support from sources which stand to benefit from a specific result. And those factors do not act independently; their interactions can also affect the validity of a conclusion. Sometimes, a thoughtful and critical doctor wonders whether available evidence can support even a maybe, much less a yes or no. So she learns the best evidence available and uses it, but never forgets that she could still be wrong.

Ioannidis also introduces a paradox: "The hotter a scientific field (with more scientific fields involved), the less likely the research findings are to be true." He argues that in a rapidly moving field, researchers are anxious to get their positive findings into print, to establish priority, while downplaying (i.e., under-reporting) negative results. This can result in an initial conclusion that either can't be duplicated, has to be modified, or is proven wrong subsequently.

So before swallowing new data completely, the good doctor recalls a familiar description of medical discovery as happening in three phases: *gee whiz*, followed by *aw shucks*, and finally *yes, but* (illustrated in the adjacent graph; this has been called the *Hype Cycle*). Since *gee whiz* is the most attractive of the three phases to scientists (as well as journalists and granting agencies), exciting results dominate the early

The Hype Cycle

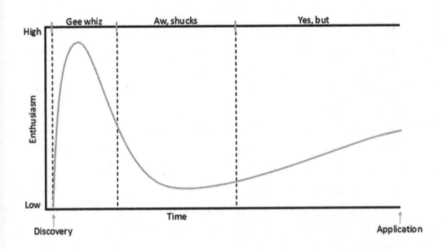

phases of discovery. But, as surely as night follows day, there are disappointments waiting in the wings that must be dealt with (*aw shucks*) before arriving at the modified expectations of clinical value (*yes, but*). The ultimate clinical value of new information, even when it turns out to be true, is almost never as great as originally claimed.

So you start to understand why the good doctor has the best chance of getting it right. Consistently attentive to new information but undazzled by extravagant claims, this doctor casts a critical eye on every source of information before using it to help you decide what to do about your health.

Randomized controlled trials are the best possible evidence, but there are many conditions for which such studies have not been done. If you have one of those conditions, how do you and your doctor decide what to do? The only choice is to resort to less reliable evidence—results of uncontrolled, non-randomized studies compared to what has been reported to happen historically, or single case reports. Even closer to the bottom of the barrel are "expert" opinions, clinical impressions, and conventional wisdom. (An old joke says that doctors tend to overvalue their clinical experience so that "in my experience . . ." is one case, "in case after case . . ." is two cases, and "in my series . . ." is three cases.) As we said earlier, opinions of TV stars, sports personalities, and other notable persons with absolutely no relevant expertise (and who are often handsomely compensated for stating their opinions on TV and in other conspicuous places) should be roundly ignored; such opinions are not evidence at all.

When the folks at the Cochrane Collaboration review a topic, they look at every level of evidence in an effort to reach some kind of expert consensus; they often fail. In forty-nine percent of 1,016 reviews in 2007, the best they could do was not yes or no but maybe; they often recommended more research. And these are the experts! For many medical conditions, there is just no clear and unequivocal answer that works for everybody. That is likely to always be true because the effects of interventions are studied in people, and people are notoriously varied and unpredictable.

What about reproducibility as a criterion for evidence? Hard scientists say to forget about any claim that cannot be duplicated by at least one more laboratory or scientist. But, assuming that most scientists don't make up results (some do and they get caught at it sooner or later), how can a scientist set up the same experiment exactly as reported by someone else and get a different answer? The good doctor knows that, unlikely as it sounds, this happens all the time. The reason is that biology, especially human biology, is so complex that it is impossible to design an experiment that doesn't have "unknown unknowns." One does the best one can to make sure that everything in the test and control groups is the same except for whatever is being tested, but one can never be absolutely sure. Human biology is not theoretical mathematics or quantum physics. These are human beings with all of the ambiguity that they bring to the table. What was the barometric pressure? What was the phase of the moon? What time of year was the study done? Where on our planet was the investigating laboratory? What was the source of reagents? For female subjects, where were they in their menstrual cycle? What was the emotional state of the test subjects? Were there critical events happening in the world at the time of the studies? Were any of the subjects survivors of intensely traumatic events either recently or in the past? Where did the test subjects live and under what circumstances? What was happening in the test subjects' families at the time of the study? Were the test subjects on some kind of fad diet? What about drugs, legal or otherwise? I'd give very long odds that the published studies your doctor reviews in an effort to decide what is right for you don't answer many of those questions. That in spite of the fact that every one of those questions could possibly affect the results of any study involving humans and so could be relevant to deciding what is right for you!

There are some other reasons why a lot of what we believe about health and disease may be wrong. One reason is that we are endlessly fascinated by observational studies—studies that link two apparently unrelated events. These make headlines almost daily. Heartburn treatments cause dementia! Coffee causes pancreatic cancer! Eating breakfast cereal causes women to give birth to more boys! Those all make good headlines and may even be based on solid observational science, but none of them is proven to be true.

Stanley Young, Assistant Director of Bioinformatics at the U.S. National Institute of Statistical Sciences, and his colleague Alan Karr identified twelve papers describing observational studies that were subsequently tested in randomized clinical trials. What do you think they discovered? Not a single one of the more critical studies agreed with the original observation, and in five of the studies the results of the definitive studies were in the opposite direction of the original report. There is a message here (alluded to in the earlier chapters). Don't trust observational studies that show associations between one variable and another, regardless of what the variables are. Remember the bucket brigade and the ebbing tide. Could be true (the bucket brigade removes water from the ocean) and true (the shoreline recedes) but unrelated.

Sometimes things happen because one thinks they should or even just because one wants them to. Of the various eponyms for these phenomena (Placebo effect, Hawthorne effect), we like *Pygmalion effect*. The reference is not to G.B. Shaw's play but to the fictional Cypriot sculptor (in Ovid's *Metamorphoses*) whose ivory carving of a woman so enraptured him that he no longer desired real women. After Pygmalion made offerings to Aphrodite wishing for a bride, "the living likeness of my ivory girl," the sculpture came to life. So the Pygmalion effect is an outcome determined solely by what was expected (or desired) of the subjects entering the study. There are plenty of examples. There are also plenty of studies showing real physiological effects of a sugar pill (Placebo effect), and definite effects resulting solely from the fact that the subjects in the study know that they are being observed (Hawthorne effect). These are not imaginings or magic tricks. These are real effects!

But are these effects that are related more to the conditions of the experiment than to the thing being tested legitimate medical evidence? If you believe something works that has no obvious scientific explanation and you do it and your condition improves, what would the good doctor who is comfortable with uncertainty say about that? She would probably say go for it! We don't understand why a lot of things work in medicine. Doctors prescribed and we took megatons of aspirin before someone discovered that it inhibited production of prostanoids, biochemicals that are major players in pain and inflammation. Doctors felt a lot better using the drug once they knew that, but aspirin didn't work any better than it ever had.

This good doctor considers herself a medical scientist, that is, she feels most confident in decisions based on sound experimental evidence. But she is also a perpetual student and never stops asking why. She realizes that important things can be learned from human experience and so she looks hard at clinical results that may lack scientific proof—pragmatic evidence. Two specific areas that interest her are eastern traditional medicine, and empirical results in everyday medical practices vis-à-vis formal clinical trials.

Eastern traditional medical practices have been used for

centuries by millions of people who believe that they are effective even though the explanations for their effects are difficult for the western medical mind to accept. A science-based physician believes that any such practices must be tested by well-designed clinical trials before they can be incorporated into the professionally sanctioned armamentarium of the practicing doctor. This is no different than is required of any medical intervention. However, the doctor comfortable with uncertainty also knows that even good clinical trials with negative results do not rule out the possibility of a therapeutic effect in some circumstances. Suppose you are doing or taking something that is clearly outside the bounds of sanctioned medical practice and you are convinced that it makes you better. If it is unlikely to do harm and there is no reason to think that it will interfere with your sanctioned treatment, the good doctor would be very likely to tell you to go ahead with it. You begin to see the healing power of uncertainty. Sometimes what's important to you is what your doctor knows she doesn't know for sure.

Pragmatic evidence also becomes an issue when there is a difference between the subjects who participate in randomized prospective clinical trials and the patients seen in actual medical practices. The very fact that design of a clinical trial requires focusing on the condition to be studied and minimizing any confounding conditions means that the people in the study may not be exactly like you or the other people who sit in doctors' offices waiting for advice.

Recognition of this problem has birthed the emerging field of *pragmatic research trials*. The reasoning is simple. Test the therapy in patients in real medical practices who have all of the confounding conditions that may affect outcomes. Include essentially everybody with the condition being studied, regardless of what else they have. The question is, are the results of the tightly controlled trial the same as results from studies in unselected patients being seen in an everyday medical practice? The pragmatic researcher might argue that if they aren't, then the data from the more rigidly controlled studies is interesting but meaningless in the real medical world.

We strongly suspect that Dr. Ioannidis would threaten apoplexy at the thought of such experiments. How does one interpret the data? What kinds of statistics can be applied to such situations? Dr. Iaonnidis would not be at all surprised if the messier experiment in the clinic failed to find the statistically significant results that the more rigidly controlled experiment claimed. The good doctor will keep abreast of these pragmatic studies, but will view them in the context of all of the other available information about your condition and will do her best to understand what the aggregated information means to you.

Try as you might to avoid it, there will always be uncertainty. All evidence-based conclusions are subject to revision as more evidence comes to light. The good doctor knows that evidence plays a vital role in health care, but she also knows that the available evidence may not be the final word.

CHAPTER 9

Information Is Not Necessarily Knowledge

Paradoxically, the more I learn about medical
problems, the less I seem to know . . .
—PHILLIP K. PETERSON, M.D., in *Get Inside Your Doctor's Head*

Don't worry very much about whether your doctor has
enough *information* about your condition. One doesn't have
to remember all that stuff anymore; it's all there and available
at the click of a mouse to anyone with a WiFi connection.
But you should worry a lot about two things: Can your
doctor critically evaluate the unfiltered deluge of information released by that mouse click, pick out the flowers
from among the garbage? And does your doctor understand
what the information means, *does she transform information into
knowledge*?

TMI (too much information), a texter's common response
to oversharing, is an appropriate comment on the state of
medical information available on the internet.

Google virtually any term you can think of that has to
do with a health-related topic of interest, and a mouse click
will flood your computer screen with thousands of hits that
purport to contain reliable information on the topic. So the
problem is not getting information. The problem is that you
can access more information than you can possibly assimilate

and that what you get is an olio of facts of varying credibility and pure fictions, each nicely presented with similar claims, equally attractive computer graphics, and equally convincing narratives. The odds of coming away from such a blind search with anything like an accurate view of the topic you were trying to understand aren't very good.

Suppose you want the latest inside scoop on how to be as sure as you can be that your new infant will not die in her sleep. You google a bunch of phrases like "Infant sleep position," "Infant co-sleeping," "pacifier sleeping," etc.; Dr. Rachel Moon, professor of pediatrics at the University of Virginia, an expert on sudden infant death syndrome (SIDS), and colleagues did precisely this search using 13 different terms. Fewer than half of the 1,300 websites that Moon et al. analyzed had information consistent with the official American Academy of Pediatrics recommendations. And a lot of the sites were carefully disguised sales pitches or appeals from special interest groups. A Mayo Clinic study several years ago concluded that medical advice about several common ailments gleaned from the internet was more likely to be either unavailable or incomplete than correct and useful. You desperately need a knowledgeable doctor's help to navigate this morass if you are to extract any accurate information. She will help you do that, but she will also warn you that getting information, even accurate information, doesn't mean that you understand the problem. Some even argue that our propensity for conflating information and knowledge creates a paradox—more *information, less understanding.*

A couple of examples may help to make the point. Suppose you are in the business of manufacturing men's suits and your production manager comes up with a brilliant idea that will dramatically enhance the bottom line. He has discovered an extensive database with detailed physical measurements of men from each major ethnic group in the U.S. Based on such measurements in one hundred thousand randomly selected men in each category, statisticians have constructed in exquisite quantitative detail a physical model of the body of the average American male of each ethnicity. This intrepid manager suggests that you manufacture only one size suit in each ethnic category perfectly fitted to the statistical models. Think how much you'll save in production costs!

What are the odds of a man entering a local shop that carries your brand and finding one of your suits that fits him? Well, the odds are certainly low and depending on how good a fit the customer insists on, the odds may be zero. As soon as you start getting feedback from retailers, that production manager will be toast. His problem was not lack of accurate information; he had information in spades. His problem was that he failed to understand what the information meant and so made a devastating mistake in applying it.

Here is another example of the difference between information and understanding that Todd Rose, director of the Mind, Brain, and Education program at Harvard, uses in his book *The End of Average*. If you wanted to know how typing speed relates to accuracy, you could gather data from all the typists you could find and make a graph of the two variables, words typed per minute versus number of mistakes per minute. You would find an inverse relationship—expert typists type faster and also make fewer mistakes than we hunt-and-peck types. However, if you want to know how to improve your typing accuracy, you would be making a big mistake to force yourself to type faster; the faster you try to type the more mistakes you will make (assuming you are not a highly skilled typist). Make a graph of your individual words per minute versus mistakes per minute and the relationship will be positive, exactly opposite the data from the expert group. Understanding the relationship between typing speed and accuracy requires that you know the circumstances. The population data do not predict an individual result.

Your doctor should know that *statistically analyzed population data don't fit any specific person.* When judged by such information, we are all misfits. The clothing industry deals with this by producing a range of sizes from which the shopper can select the one that fits best, recognizing that the fit won't be perfect. Likewise, there is usually a range of options in a given medical situation and choices are made that take into account characteristics of the specific patient. However, the thinking doctor understands that even so, the fit may not be as good as it can be, and so she is constantly looking for anything about you that could cause you to respond differently from the subjects studied in clinical trials. Population studies rigorously done and carefully analyzed are critically important to your health care, but a doctor who knows and understands those studies will realize that their value is in demonstrating interventions' effects or lack thereof in groups of your fellow humans and not necessarily in how precisely they predict what will happen to you.

The good doctor knows that the same information may be crucial in one situation and useless in another. For example, she understands the difference between practicing *public health* and practicing *medicine.*

The public health practitioner relies on data from large populations to implement policies aimed at improving overall health outcomes for a population. Success or failure can be measured by whether or not the targeted outcome improves. Count the bodies (or whatever) before and after implementing the policy, tote up the data, and do the statistics. There are many important public health successes. Fewer people get arbovirus infections when mosquito populations are controlled. Tooth decay decreases when public water supplies are fluorinated. The incidence of thyroid goiters goes down when iodine is added to table salt. The incidence and consequences of several infectious diseases and environment- or behavior-related health problems improve when the public health people aim aggressive programs at things like clean water, flush toilets, and cigarette smoking. The good doctor encourages her patients to respond to public health campaigns that promote immunizations, smoking cessation, healthy diets, etc.

But, the public health practitioner treats large aggregates of people and addresses health issues that many individuals share—the most good for the most people. The medical doctor's job is to deal with people one by one and each one she faces is different from everyone else in potentially important ways; every one of her patients is a one-off. Your doctor's responsibility is to help you to be healthier and to get you back to good health as quickly as possible when you get sick.

She knows that what the available information means to your situation may be very different from what it means to the public health policy maker. You may be a real outlier when measured against the general population, or even a subpopulation of people with a problem similar to yours. You can't make yourself type faster and expect fewer mistakes, no matter what happens in the typing world at large. You and your doctor need to figure out where you are on the spectrum of possibilities and what course of action is most likely to benefit you. The good doctor values the experts' recommendations based on what happens in large groups of people and knows that applying that knowledge to unique human beings may require some flexibility. That's why this doctor is open to the whole range of possibilities. She knows that the essence of understanding is knowing what she doesn't know for sure, and she is prepared to use that ignorance to help you, unique individual N of 1 that you are, to be as healthy as you can be.

How can you tell if your doctor is a *good doctor*, not just a nice, friendly person with good people skills? Well, there are two parts to that question: How does your doctor stack up in the larger world of doctoring? And how well-served is your health in this specific doctor-patient partnership?

Driven largely by the needs of health care managers and funding sources to measure productivity, efficiency, and quality of care, a lot of effort is expended searching for metrics, things that can be measured and expressed in numbers that accurately reflect whether or not a doctor is good at what she does. This is harder than you might think. True, some things can be measured—blood sugar and related biochemicals, blood pressure, blood cholesterol levels, etc.—and such measurements in all of the patients in a doctor's practice give some notion of success for those specific health outcomes in that group of patients. But if we must have metrics (numbers) then we'll be judging how good a doctor is from the limited number of things that are readily measurable. For example, none of the doctor rating systems (there are several) include a measure of misdiagnosis, which is surely a critical measure of a doctor's skills. The National Academy of Medicine says that misdiagnosis, arriving at the wrong conclusion for what is causing a person's illness, is not a rare problem; somewhere between 10 and 25 percent of diagnoses are wrong. One study published in 2012 concludes that more than forty thousand patients die annually in this country's intensive care units as a direct result of a wrong diagnosis. You doctor may have all the right boxes checked off on the list of measurable things and still be less effective than you would like.

And a lot of undigitized things influence how well a doctor's patients do—socioeconomics, severity of illness, mental and emotional capacity, etc.—so when the numbers are added up, they may or may not look good depending on some intangibles that are difficult to account for. It is even possible that the noblest doctors wind up with poor ratings based on the numbers because of whom they choose to serve. Those numbers are information and we should pay some attention to them, but we should not forget that information is not knowledge. If you really want to know how good your doctor is, you'll need to look beyond the numbers.

In spite of acknowledged flaws in any numbers-based

rating system, the health care managers continue to insist that such ratings are essential for making doctors accountable and improving the value of health care. *If you can't measure it you can't manage it* goes the old business adage with an intuitive appeal that captivates the suits. The idea has even found its way into U.S. law! The Affordable Care Act requires the Center for Medicare and Medicaid Services (CMS) to "make publicly available . . . information on physician performance that provides comparable information on quality and patient experience measures." Beginning with a web site called *Physician Compare*, the feds are well on their way to giving us a doctor rating system. Well, what's wrong with that? Doctors should surely be accountable for what they do, and we need some way to know if we are getting what we are paying for medicine-wise.

There's nothing wrong with getting the available numbers and collating the data in a way that we can grasp. The big flaw in this approach is mistaking information for understanding. The conscientious doctor will pay close attention to her numerical scores, however they turn out to be developed and expressed. She will use those numbers to improve the things that she does that can be digitized. You ought to look at the numbers too; they are information. However, your doctor and you will value what she does, judge how good a doctor she is, from your personal experiences in this health care relationship—How healthy are you? When you get sick, how quickly do you return to health? How often and how badly does your doctor get it wrong and how does she deal with such mistakes? Don't count on others' opinions either; Press-Ganey scores, a commonly used measure of patient satisfaction, are, again, *information*, but they are not *understanding*. If a doctor refuses to prescribe antibiotics for a bad cold or some other unproven remedy hawked by a guy wearing surgical scrubs on TV, a disappointed patient may give her bad Press-Ganey scores precisely because she did the right thing—a bad score for a good doctor. Such scores may have little to do with your personal experience with your doctor and even less to do with how good she is at her chosen profession.

But still, argue proponents of digitized medicine, if enough health-related things could be measured, it should be possible (given the robustness of increasingly muscular computers) to integrate all that information into numbers that accurately describe the quality of your care. The problem, these folks would say, is that too few things can be measured and so the major advances to come will be in measurement technology and computer programs for integrating information. Give computers enough information and clever enough algorithms and they can transform information into knowledge.

The current boom in wearable sensors that translate what's happening in your body into numbers is an example of this approach. And emerging technologies will expand the potential of such devices beyond what we can imagine now. According to Gary Wolf, author of *Quantified Self*, we may be able, before long, to monitor in real time, in quantitative terms, "sleep, exercise, sex, food, mood, location, alertness, productivity, even spiritual well-being." New measurements are being added to the list at a dizzying pace. Wolf says, "more than thirty thousand new personal tracking projects are started by users every month." It may well be that the coincidence of tiny electronic sensors, powerful smart phones, social media, and the cloud will enable construction of your *quantified self.* We will learn a lot about human health from such attempts. They may even shed some new light on the challenge of relating population data to your uniquely personal condition and evaluating your doctor's performance.

The numbers game is enticing to doctors as well as patients. Like Thomas Gradgrind in the Dickens novel *Hard Times*, when faced with the ambiguity that is inevitable in human conditions, both we and our doctors are tempted to plead, "Fact, fact, fact!" The American Heart Association's website encourages you to "Know Your Health Numbers"—weight, body mass index, blood sugar, blood pressure, cholesterol, maybe even hemoglobin A1c (a diabetes index) and C reactive protein (a measure of inflammation).

Numbers sound like something solid that you can rely on, but it's not so simple. If you Google *know your numbers* you'll get ten pages of hits luring you to a variety of programs with cleverly designed web pages. Some of these have been accused of "non-evidence-based fear mongering." And you don't want to lay awake nights worrying about your hemoglobin A1c or your C-reactive protein unless those numbers have a personal meaning to you. Losing sleep will likely make the numbers worse, threatening a spiral of mutually reinforcing unhealthy results.

So you'll need help sorting out the best numbers-based program for you. And you'll also need help prioritizing the numbers, evaluating their accuracy, and understanding how your behavior influences them. If you decide to get into the numbers game by yourself, you're likely to run into trouble. A good doctor can help.

But the good doctor also knows that what's best for you isn't always determined by the numbers. *Information is not understanding!* If you fall down the entranceway stairs in your condo and break your leg, this doctor knows that you'll want to get it taken care of as fast as possible. She'll see that you get a proper cast, adequate pain medication, a walking cast as soon as possible to free you from the crutches, and the cast removed after the minimum required number of days. However, she also knows that if you are a cross-country skier and break your leg, you may want something quite different. You'll want to be free of pain of course. You'll want to get rid of the crutches and the sooner you can get rid of that pesky cast, the happier you'll be. But, what you really, really want is to be back on your skies schussing across a pristine snowfield inhaling the brisk winter morning air. As far as you're concerned, the value of your attempts to be healthy is tied directly to how much they advance you toward what you really, really want. If leaving the cast on a few more days and continuing with the crutches, or even dealing with some additional pain, will get you back on your skis faster, then you'll probably go for it. And you'll go for it with this doctor's blessing. She understands.

The people who study behavior talk about *value driven planning.* That's where you plan to use your resources to do the things you value most, starting at the top of the list. Some people do a better job of taking care of their health if they approach it that way. While tracking numbers may make a lot of us behave in healthier ways, for some of us, what feels important can be a more potent motivator than numbers. If you can realize the things you value most about your health, the numbers may take care of themselves. You might practice yoga or meditation. The idea of mindfulness might appeal to you and mindful eating may be the most effective way for you to control your diet. You might find the time for long walks in the park, or time in the early mornings to sit in the garden and listen to the birds awaken. Your doctor should keep track of your numbers and see that you pay attention to the important ones. But she will realize that *you* may be more value driven to do whatever you need to do to be healthy. The thoughtful doctor knows your numbers, she has the *information*, but she also *understands* what they mean to you.

CHAPTER 10

The Good, the Bad, and the Ugly of Statistics

When we use single numbers to estimate uncertain future outcomes . . . we are not just usually wrong, but are consistently wrong.
—from Harry Markowitz's foreword to *The Flaw of Averages: Why We
Underestimate Risk in the Face of Uncertainty* by Sam L. Savage

Here's the good doctor's problem with statistics. Statistical
significance is the virtually universal criterion that medical
doctors and scientists use to determine what is true. But the
good doctor knows that statistics are perfectly capable of
lying. Statisticians tacitly admit that. The American writer
Darrel Huff even wrote a DIY manual on the subject that
he titled *How to Lie With Statistics,* the best-selling statistics
book of the second half of the twentieth century.

Statistics are about *probabilities* (how likely something is
to be true or not) and the magic number is 0.05 (or 5 percent). If results have less than a five percent chance of being
wrong ($p<0.05$; *statistically significant* in the jargon) then
they are deemed likely to be true. But a probability of 0.05
means that there is a one in twenty chance that the results are
totally random, not true at all. And how does your doctor
know if you're among the one in twenty for whom the truth
is different than what the statistics say? Of course she doesn't
know until she learns everything she possibly can about you

and maybe not until after some diagnostic and therapeutic trial and error. The problem is that statistics are meaningless for an N of 1; and you, I, and the other seven or so billion of our kind are each an N of 1.

One of us (MMEJ) practiced for many years as a cancer surgeon. His conversation with a patient newly diagnosed with a serious cancer might have gone something like this:

Patient: *Well, doc, what are my chances of beating this thing?*

MMEJ: *Your chances of surviving this are either 0 or 100 percent.*

Patient: *What do you mean? Can't you give me a number, some kind of odds?*

MMEJ: *If you want to know what percent of a large group of people with this cancer will survive it, I will of course give you a number. But for you personally, it's all or none. You will either survive it or you won't. So let's be positive and assume that you're a survivor.*

Patient: *I'm not sure whether I ought to feel optimistic or depressed.*

MMEJ: *Given the only alternative, don't you think it makes the most sense to assume you're going to beat it?*

Patient: *Maybe so, doc. Maybe so.*

What this imaginary patient was told was true, but having convinced him that he and his doctor should set out a course of treatment assuming the best possible outcome, then what?

None of the three major therapies for cancer—surgery, radiation, or drugs either separately or in some combination—is without serious collateral damage. So how do the doctor and the patient decide on a treatment that has the best chance of succeeding while doing the least harm?

Well, in spite of the argument that statistical analysis of population studies may not be relevant to an individual patient, we have to start somewhere, and so we start with the one size suit, the statistical results of rigorously conducted and analyzed studies of groups of patients with a similar disease. A one size suit is, after all, better than no suit at all.

That's a starting place, but where do we go from there? Sorry, but a few more words about statistics are necessary since that is how most folks go about measuring the value of evidence.

Most studies of effects of interventions in groups of patients are analyzed using *frequency-based statistics*—means, medians, confidence limits—all of the numbers from individual patients condensed into uber-numbers that describe the whole population and carry the weight of statistical authenticity; $p < 0.05$=probably true, $p > 0.05$=maybe not. But these numbers don't apply directly to individuals even in the study group, much less to the patient sitting in a doctor's office examining room anxiously awaiting advice about what to do and feeling very much alone. Some statisticians have taken on this problem and tried to expand their craft to deal with how information from groups can be used to inform a specific circumstance. Those efforts started around the middle of the eighteenth century.

In addition to coming to grips with her reservations about

statistics mentioned above, somewhere along her way, the good doctor also met the elusive statistician, philosopher, and, judging from an alleged portrait, somewhat overweight and dour Presbyterian minister, Rev. Thomas Bayes of Tunbridge Wells, Kent, England. Rev. Bayes was born circa 1701 and died at the age of fifty-nine having never published the work that is his major legacy. His notes on what came to be called *Bayes theorem* were published two years after his death by his friend Richard Price in the *Philosophical Transactions of the Royal Society of London*. The article was titled, "An Essay towards solving a Problem in the Doctrine of Chances" and the ideas described in the article gave rise to an entire field of what is still known as *Bayesian statistics*.

The basic idea of Bayesian statistics is that the likelihood of a specific thing happening, the statisticians' probability, is influenced by a number of factors in addition to previous group experiences and that probability changes as more information becomes available. There is a school of thought that this way of interpreting medically related information is closer to being accurate and is more useful in practice than the more commonly used frequency-based approach.

Without dealing with the math, here are a couple of illustrations of how it works. Computer scientist, engineer, and educator Kevin Boone uses the simple illustration of picking a probable winner of a two horse race—he calls the horses Fleetfoot and Dogmeat. The horses have raced head to head twelve times in the past; Fleetfoot won seven of those races. Seems easy, bet on Fleetfoot. But it turns out that on four of those occasions it was raining and on the rainy days Dogmeat won three of the four races. So if it's raining on the day of the race, bet on Dogmeat (ignoring the poor animal's unfortunate name). If it's sunny, put your money on Fleet-foot. *When additional factors are taken into account the predicted outcome may differ from that predicted by the overall data from the entire experience.*

But the implications of additional information are not always so obvious. Consider the Monty Hall problem. You are a contestant on the quiz show *Let's Make a Deal* and Mr. Hall, the show's host, tells you that two of three closed doors hide a goat and the third hides a car. You are to guess which one has the car and you choose door number one. Before finalizing your choice, Mr. Hall opens door number two revealing a goat and gives you the opportunity to either stick with your original guess or change it to door number three. What choice gives you the better chance of revealing the car?

Here's how the reasoning goes. The probability of your original choice of door number one being correct is one in three, unaffected by the new information. The probably of your original guess being wrong is then two in three. Since now there is only one other choice and your original guess is more likely to be wrong than to be right, you should change your guess to door number three. That may require some digesting, but *the point is that new information may change probabilities of a given outcome in unexpected ways.*

But what does this have to do with how the good doctor would deal with her cancer patient? Well, she would start with the available population data, but then she would look carefully at this specific person. How old is he? Does he have any other health problems? What is his race or ethnic group, his socioeconomic status? Does he have a personal support system that he can rely on? Where does he live? Does he have readily available transportation? What are his health related beliefs? Is there a family history of cancer and if so how was it treated and what was the outcome? And even, yes, what are the relevant base sequences in his genome DNA? In short, this doctor gathers every bit of information about the person that has any chance of influencing how likely he is to accept and respond to a given treatment. Then, what about the cancer—the cell type, the clinical stage (caught early and still localized, widely spread to other sites in the body, or somewhere in between), and perhaps the cancer's genotype as well? All of those variables and any other information that indicates possible effects of the personal characteristics of this patient and the specifics of his cancer are taken into account in designing an initial treatment plan.

Bayesian probability also changes as new information becomes available; if it's raining on race day we just have to grit our teeth and put our money on Dogmeat. So this patient's initial responses to a regimen, new discoveries about the biology of his kind of cancer, and other changes in his condition or circumstances may alter his prognosis and his therapy. One of University of Minnesota professor Phillip Peterson's ten rules for doctoring is: "If What You're Doing Doesn't Seem to Be Working, Think About Doing Something Else." Another of his rules is: "If What You're Doing Seems to Be Working, Think About Continuing It."

Although perhaps less than thoroughly versed in the history, theory, and mathematics of Bayesian statistics, a doctor who has made peace with uncertainty does think like a

Bayesean. The very fact that predicting outcomes is complex and that such probabilities are not static but are subject to change based on what happens in real time requires that the entire spectrum of possibilities remains open from beginning to end of a person's illness. The responsible doctor knows this and stays in touch with all the possibilities. It also means that if "evidence" means the results of clinical trials analyzed by frequency-based statistics, then relying on evidence as the sole basis for deciding on therapy may limit the chances of getting the best results in any specific case.

Living in this twenty-first century, it is impossible to avoid attempts to convert all problems to number problems. There is a prevailing notion that most of the human dilemma will eventually be made tractable by the truly scary power of the computer, and medicine is not an exception. Granted, Stanford and Cambridge professor Sam Savage's *Flaw of Averages* exposes the naiveté of imagining that a *single* number will magically transfer all critical decisions from the human brain to Watson or who(what)ever. But if we knew all the numbers and how they influence each other, that might be possible; it would just be a matter of working out the math. And given a marketplace teeming with devices for measuring stuff related to health that are not tethered to a laboratory or a doctor, is it possible that even the subjective part of diagnosis and treatment, the *art of medicine,* might become essentially a machine activity with little need for flesh-and-blood professionals?

There is a rising chorus of people who favor moving health care in that direction. (*New York Times* physician writer, Abigail Zuger, wonders whether such people are practicing medicine on a different planet than the one where she works.) A serious challenge to this approach is converting each step of the process into formulas, equations, and, ultimately, numbers, what has been called the *digitization of health care.*

There are mathematical approaches to analyzing how decisions emerge from complex interactions among people; one approach is called *game theory.* This is not game as in parlor game. This is serious stuff. Game theory has been used to analyze the Cuban missile crisis, the Viet Nam peace negotiations, the Watergate scandal, and even the existence of God. You can't get much more serious than that! There are several Nobel laureates in economics among the game theorists and the species is also to be found comfortably ensconced in the ranks of sociologists, psychologists, astronomers, and evolutionary biologists. Maybe game theory can rescue medical decision making and models of medical consultation from the murky netherworld of subjectivity and intuition.

There have been efforts to do just that. For example, Carolyn Tarrant and her associates at the University of Leicester examined the utility of several game theory models with snappy names—the Prisoner's Dilemma game, the Assurance game, the Centipede game—to analyze medical consultations. Others are doing similar work in an effort to understand and predict how medical decisions are made with the ultimate goal of making it a numbers game and delegating responsibility to an algorithm. No doubt a lot will be learned about how people behave in a medical setting from the game theorists, but the ultimate goal may be elusive. Perhaps some processes can be digitized, but people tend to be pretty determinedly analog. The effectiveness and efficiency of health care will benefit from efforts of the game theorists, but it seems unlikely that they will seriously threaten your doctor's place in the care of the real person that is you.

Archimedes might be a more serious threat. Not the ancient Greek mathematician who ran into the streets naked from his bath shouting *Eureka! Eureka!* upon discovering that the displacement of water could be used to determine the volume of an irregular object. That guy did a lot of interesting things, but we mean, "Archimedes: An Analytical Tool for Improving the Quality and Efficiency of Health Care," the brainchild of Kaiser Permanente's David M. Eddy, who may have been the first person to use the term *evidence based medicine*.

Dr. Eddy opens an article describing his brainchild this way: "The practice of medicine has become extraordinarily complex, and it promises to become even more complex as the pace of innovation accelerates." As he goes on to describe his model, we are thinking, "You can say that again." Digitizing health care, as Bette Davis said about getting old, *ain't no place for sissies.* A fundamental complexity is what Joe Loscalzo and colleagues have called *network medicine.* It's not just that there are probably millions of bits of information to deal with, but that each of those million bits interacts with all of the other millions of bits and those interactions have to be accounted for if anything useful is to come out of the effort. But computers are capable of dealing with mindboggling complexity if you can give them the numbers, so Dr. Eddy, who is both a physician and an information expert, had a go at it; Archimedes is the result.

Dr. Eddy and his colleagues scoured the literature for the

relevant basic research, epidemiological studies, and clinical trials. They built a three-part model: a model of human physiology; care process models; and models of system resources, personnel, facilities, equipment, costs, etc. Then they wrote over two hundred (we didn't count them) equations describing the interactions of all these variables, fed them into the computer, and flipped the start switch.

Does Archimedes work? Well, it can produce results of virtual clinical trials that very closely simulate the results of actual trials. More needs to be done, but if it were possible to do clinical trials *in silico* instead of *in vivo*, sparing living people the inconvenience and risks of such studies, that would be pretty amazing.

Archimedes has been acquired by Evidera, a "health care modeling and analytics organization." They claim that "the company enables people to combine real-world health care data and simulation data to create compelling and actionable evidence used in individual health care decision making, as well as in populations, with applications in health and economic outcomes research, policy creation, and clinical trial design and operations." Time will tell whether those promises will be kept and how they color the practice of medicine. Although the thinking doctor isn't holding her breath, she will keep a close eye on Archimedes.

So, how does your doctor, knowing a good bit about how science comes by and interprets numbers, consider your personal health? Will she see you as that unique N of 1 for whom the general experiences of humanity may not always apply? Or will she lump you together with the statistical crowd, confidently relying on those general human experiences to tell her how to keep you healthy or get you well? Should we all start preparing ourselves for the brave new world of digitized medicine while doctors look for another job? Or can we have it both ways? Can you and your doctor preserve your individuality as a critical factor in your care while still benefitting from all of the quantitative stuff?

Stephen Jay Gould's fascinating essay "The Median Isn't the Message," which we mentioned earlier, speaks elegantly to this quandary. He was diagnosed with a disease that the literature describes as incurable with a median survival time from diagnosis of five months. He died twenty years later of an unrelated condition. What was his secret?

Dr. Gould believed that at least part of his secret lay in his understanding of statistics and how they applied to his specific circumstance. Not a fatalist by nature, he was unwilling to accept the conclusion that he had only five months to live. He knew that a median survival time meant that half of the people with the disease lived longer than that. Further he discovered that survivals of patients with his disease were "right skewed," that is a few people, although not many, lived a lot longer than the median—years longer. So Dr. Gould set about to see where he fit on this oddly right skewed survival curve. He concluded that there were several reasons to think that his niche on the curve was way out to the right on the longevity tail—he was young, he was getting excellent medical care, his disease was diagnosed early, and he was enthusiastic about the future. During the ensuing twenty years, Dr. Gould made major contributions to our understanding of the world and inspired two generations of

Harvard students to better understand and care about that world.

It is possible that you are a statistic but not a common one, that you have a number but that it falls somewhere outside the boundaries of conventional thinking. All the more reason to find yourself a doctor who can think conventionally, but is perfectly comfortable with unconventionality when the occasion calls for it.

CHAPTER 11

Don't Believe Everything You Read, No Matter Where You Read It

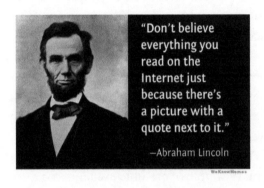

"Don't believe everything you read on the Internet just because there's a picture with a quote next to it."

—Abraham Lincoln

The good doctor doesn't need this meme to convince her of its message. She learned somewhere early in her education to be suspicious of claimed truths, especially those lacking any convincing evidence. And although she depends heavily on reputable scientific sources, this doctor knows that even highly respected science journals, her primary source of medical information, occasionally, in spite of their best efforts, wind up publishing things that turn out to be untrue, and once in a while they fail to publish potentially important and valid discoveries. While not a cynic, she rarely takes information at face value, no matter the source, and she always remembers that she may not be seeing the entire picture.

In 1914 American writer and explorer of anomalous phenomena Charles Fort published a work titled *The Book of the Damned*. He was convinced that mainstream scientists were slaves to current trends, excluding (*damning*) observations that didn't fit their preconceptions. In *The Book of the Damned* he expounded his theory and discussed a number of truly strange phenomena that he concluded were damned to obscurity without a fair and objective hearing by the arrogant conventionality of popular science. While the doctor who accepts uncertainty is no *Fortean*—those students of strange phenomena who are ready to believe almost anything—she recognizes that Fort's idea may sometimes have merit. Subjective factors do sometimes affect, at least for the time being, what science gets published and thus what *facts* become generally accepted.

For American medicine, as for all of western medicine, the primary source of credible evidence for or against a given intervention is the published medical literature. If research is not published, preferably in a reputable scientific journal, then the only people who know about it are the scientists who did the work and perhaps their friends and family and the bartender at the after-work hangout behind the hospital. Whether work is published is decided by the researchers who do it; they must analyze the data, do the statistics, and write the manuscript. But decisions about publication also involve the journal editors and a select group of usually two or three presumed experts in the area who review the manuscript and give it a thumbs up or down; that is called peer review. This process is not perfect; there are multiple opportunities for slips twixt the metaphorical cup and lip. The thinking doctor is very familiar with this system (at various times in her career she was probably both rewarded and punished by it) and she always remembers that the *available* information may not be the whole story.

For one thing, while well-done studies with negative results are seriously considered for publication by editors of highly regarded medical journals, they and their peer reviewers tend to be more excited by positive results. And academic careers depend heavily on publishing original research in well-regarded journals. Negative experimental outcomes can languish in lab notebooks, never even converted into a manuscript. Even if an industrious post doc gins up enough energy to write up an elegantly done but thoroughly negative study, it can be hard to make it through a highly regarded journal's editorial and peer reviews, and the return on the necessary investment of time and energy needed to find a lesser journal that will publish it may not be enough to make it worth the trouble. Should the negative studies find their way into some less than stellar journal, they will have a limited impact on conventional understanding of the subject because they will be less exposed to and less respected by influential people than the positive studies that are discussed *ad infinitum* by the elite readers of higher impact publications.

So, there is a body of research with negative results that no one knows about and that is not considered when compiling the evidence for or against a given intervention. Your doctor just doesn't know a lot about what doesn't work or even what works sometimes under some circumstances in some people but doesn't work in other situations. This is scientifically sound research which too rarely gets into the body of medical evidence because of the bias of a publication process favoring positive results that are not too far afield from conventional thinking.

And—a sad commentary on the whole scientific enterprise—occasionally there are scientists who lie and cheat and are clever enough at it to get their "work" published in respected journals. Some people think that this behavior is getting worse and blame it on increasing academic pressures to publish. There are academic pressures, but they don't excuse dishonesty. Pressures to publish may smoke out the scoundrels among us, but lying and cheating are failures of character, not faults of a system.

How rampant is dishonesty in medical research? One measure, which no doubt underestimates the problem, is the number of articles that are published and subsequently retracted. *Retraction Watch*, which follows numbers of and reasons for retractions, estimates that scientific articles are retracted at a rate of one per day and that the rate is increasing. Surprisingly, the very journals that your doctor ought to be able to trust, the ones from which articles are most often cited by publishing scientists, are the ones that retract the most articles! The good doctor knows that you can't really trust any one source, that figuring out what is right in a given circumstance requires gathering all of the information one can find and assembling as complete a picture as possible with all of the materials in hand.

Not only are negative results often unavailable, but the influence of positive results is also often exaggerated. Studies with positive results are: more likely to be published quickly; more likely to generate multiple publications; more likely to be published in a "high impact" journal; more likely to be cited by other investigators; and more likely to be published in English. Those are all reasons why experts especially value positive results when they sit down to weigh the evidence. So the experts' evidence, a distillation of the available information, could be distorted by unknown negative results and by over-valued positive results.

Does this actually happen at the real-world interface of the known and unknown amid the babble and clatter of scientific discovery? The answer is probably yes, but you don't have to take our word for it.

"Published results of scientific investigations are not a representative sample of results of all scientific studies," write Simon Fraser University School of Computing Science investigators T. D. Sterling, W. L. Rosenbaum, and J. J. Weinkam in a 1995 article in *The American Statistician*. They found biases toward publishing studies that showed statistically significant positive results in eleven major journals. This has two bad effects. One is that investigators, having no way to know about unpublished data, keep doing experiments that others, maybe several others, have proven don't work. That wastes money and even more valuable resources—the time, energy and enthusiasm of medical investigators.

The second, follow-on effect hinges on the words *statistically significant*. That requirement means that smaller studies and those with less significant results—suppose your p value was 0.06—are unlikely to see the light of day. This in spite of the fact that everybody knows that $p < 0.05$ is a completely arbitrary threshold for significance and that results with higher p values may be just as true as those that happen to make the passing statistical grade. So some things that might actually work go unreported, which means lost opportunities.

So how much of the information from clinical trials gets published and so is widely available? Probably around half. That figure is astounding, but it may be true. We'll explain why we say it may be true below, but think for a minute about what this means. Your doctor knows that the results of maybe half of the trials of treatments that she is contemplating recommending to you may have gone unreported in the literature. Such studies would have had minimal influence on the expert panels that developed guidelines, or on the Cochrane Collaboration's reviewers, or on the meta-analysts. Faced with a specific person with a specific problem, how does the good doctor go about making a decision? First of all, she carefully assesses the available evidence in the context of what she knows about you. After all, even imperfect evidence is the factual basis for making health decisions, and the good doctor values facts. She also knows that there may be an unknown number of unreported studies that were either negative or inconclusive and that the reported positive studies may be over-valued by the experts who decide on the evidence. Given all of that, how does your doctor figure out what is most likely to help you get or stay well? Sooner or later you and she will have to deal with uncertainty.

What about the claim that half of the clinical trials data is never published? How can we know for sure since we are dealing with (if we have our Rumsfeldisms straight) an *unknown known,* that is, things that are known by someone but not by us? Well, in the case of clinical trials, one can get a pretty good idea because of the foresight of our federal government in establishing by law in 2008 the database known as ClinicalTrials.gov.

The U.S. Food and Drug Administration Act obligates clinical investigators to post the results of all clinical trials of Food and Drug Administration-approved drugs on ClinicalTrials.gov within a year of completing the study. So, on March 27, 2012, Parisian clinical epidemiologist Carolina Riveros and her colleagues searched that database for the results of randomized controlled trials. For a random sample of six hundred of those trials, they also searched PubMed, a separate database that lists essentially all medical publications. You've already guessed where the 50 percent number comes from. Of the six hundred trials reported in ClinicalTrials.gov, only 297 were reported in a published article. And it gets worse. In 202 studies for which there were published articles, adverse and serious adverse events were significantly under reported in the published articles compared to the government database; apparently the legal obligation outweighs the moral one . . . disappointing.

So, the available medical information may be biased toward positive results and against negative findings. Apart from complicating a doctor's efforts to help her patients decide what is right for them, does it really matter? Yes, it matters. It can matter a lot!

While we have no inside information about what drives British medical researcher Andrew Wakefield or about the review process of the prestigious British medical journal *The Lancet*, we, and the rest of the world, know now that the 1998 *Lancet* paper claiming that childhood vaccinations cause autism was bogus. The editors of *The Lancet* know that too; they retracted the article in 2010, rather late in the wake of a deluge of scientific, professional and social criticism of the motives, performance, and reporting of Wakefield's studies. If it wasn't a less than healthy fascination with dramatic positive results, then we have no idea why *The Lancet* accepted this article, but we would bet the farm that, before that article appeared, an identical study concluding that there was no link between vaccination and autism would have been soundly rejected!

We earlier referred to Wakefield et al.'s *Lancet* paper as "the holy text" of the anti-vaccine movement, a movement with real consequences. More susceptible children sets the stage for the reappearance of diseases that vaccination programs had largely eliminated from this country. The multistate measles epidemic in 2015 is a dramatic illustration. Medical researchers' and their journals' relentless pursuit of positive and interesting results sometimes has serious consequences that are not good, and once the erroneous information genie is out there it is hard to force the wily rascal back into the bottle.

Recognizing the potential and real downside of publication bias in medicine, scientists have given some serious thought to possible remedies. Here are some possibilities that have been considered: link research funding for clinical studies to quantity of publications (since most researchers have more negative than positive data, this might get some more of the negative stuff into circulation); continue efforts to create a culture among investigators, academic institutions, and elite journals that values well done and definitive negative studies (culture change is hard, good luck); create negative results sections in medical journals; and create new journals specifically for publishing negative results.

David Alcantara Parra, Spanish chemist and nanoscientist, created the *All Results Journals* (ARJournals) specifically intended to "make use of all the data that go unreported within the scientific community." Building on the premise that "failure is as important in science as in other aspects of life," the *Journal of Negative Results in Biomedicine (JNRBM)* was launched in 2002 with Harvard Professor of Developmental Biology Bjorn Olsen as its editor. The focus of the journal is in ecology and evolutionary biology, but there could be value in emulating it in fields more directly relevant to the practice of medicine.

The good doctor knows all of this. She knows how important the published literature is and studies it religiously, but she also knows that like most things that humans do, the literature is not perfect. So how does she go about getting as close as possible to a reasonably good look at a complete and accurate picture?

Were you to barge into the office unannounced, you might well find the good doctor staring intently at a computer screen. She is what we will call a *discriminating web surfer* (to be clearly distinguished from the more numerous *naïve, recreational,* or *gullible* varieties of the species). This doctor uses all available tools (there are many, e.g. WebMD, Up-To-Date, even when desperate maybe Google) to flatten her medical world. She values published information but does not hesitate to cast a wide net in her efforts to understand the whole picture; in the computer age, absent barriers of geography or time, she can cast an enormously wide net. Of course she realizes that a wide net collects a lot of garbage (she is no fan of bizarre conspiracy theories, and stories of alien forces or political intrigue don't excite her), which is where her powers of discrimination become indispensable. That is why you need her help.

A lot of the negative results and some of the less statistically significant but positive results that didn't make it into the mainstream medical literature are retrievable from the cloud, and those results may fill in some details of the picture outlined in the published literature. That is, if one can, like the famous detective, "recognize, out of a number of facts, which are incidental and which are vital."

A thinking doctor knows that contributions to the internet are often not critically curated, so she starts by sorting out the needles of facts from the haystack of fictions. If you try to do this all by yourself at home, you are sure to make mistakes; we are all more vulnerable to the influence of misinformation than we would like to admit. This good doctor spent a lot of years learning the stuff one needs to know to pick out what is true and important. That's one reason why insurance companies pay doctors. No thoughtful doctor gets her legal advice from bartenders, relatives, or anyone else who posts their ruminations on the internet; she consults a lawyer. You are wise to deal with your health care needs similarly; consult a doctor.

Only a fraction of what fills the widely cast net of even the most dedicated and discriminating web surfer will be actual data. There are a lot of opinions, musings, theories (too often ill-founded and almost always untested), confabulations, inane comments on this or that, the stuff of the haystack. But this doctor is looking for data.

"Data! Data! Data!" Sherlock Holmes cried, "I can't make bricks without clay."

In medicine, data with a capital D is on the way. It is said and published in multiple places that a sea change is afoot that will not just rewrite the rules, but will make health care an entirely new game. Will the imminent age of big data run contemplative doctors out of business? Probably not, but their job and how they do it will change a lot.

There will surely be seismic changes in how fast information gets out and what can be done with it. Digital visionaries writing in *The Fourth Paradigm* imagine a time of *health care singularity*, meaning real time generation, processing, analysis, communication, and integration of data related to human health. Enormous amounts of data, assembled into functional networks and available as interactive models, could give the future doctor an entirely new set of tools for accessing and interpreting research results. Journals as we know them could become relics of historical interest but of little practical use.

And the age of big data for health care is imminent, ushered in by the deluge of medical information being collected and stored, coupled with quantum advances in the technology that promise to convert those data into understanding. There are a lot of things still to be worked out, but the potential boggles the mind. Might the time come when you and your doctor can get to all of your health-related data instantly, no matter where it was collected, in a single place in the cloud? That would be a major advance. But then if your data were put in the context of the relevant data from all of your fellow humans and all of the available research on the subject you're worried about, analyzed, and the implications spelled out for you, your doctor might start to get a little nervous about your need for her. You would have not just the clay but the bricks already made.

Well, you may have the bricks, but you still haven't built the house and you can't do that alone, even with the help of your trusty computer. The digitization of medicine, when done, will dramatically increase the availability, accuracy, and efficiency of health care, but it won't eliminate the need for flesh-and-blood professionals. Roles will change. Doctors will need some new skills and will need to know some stuff that isn't critical in the present health care world. But no matter how perfectly the digital world works, we human beings will still be analog; it is the nature of the beast. We will always need a wise, knowledgeable, and caring partner to help us navigate the process, and our need for the healing touch of a human hand will not go away.

PART IV

Some Things to Expect from Your Doctor

CHAPTER 12

Your Story Is Front and Center—
Narrative-Based Medicine

Scientific thinking might be defined as learning to distinguish the
exception from the rule. I'd have a hard time entrusting my health to
someone who didn't know the difference.

—Stan Polanski

Ms. Sydney Blasingame (not her real name) was ninety-eight
years old and still preferred to be addressed as Miss Syd. Her
primary school students had called her that for many years
and she treasured the memories of those years. Miss Syd was
doing pretty well for her age, but she did have a little high
blood pressure and her heart wasn't pumping quite as well
as it did in her more vigorous past. For many years, Miss
Syd had been cared for by a senior physician in the clinic of
a large university medical center. Her doctor, a professor in
the medical school, decided to take a well-earned sabbatical
leave to study some new laboratory techniques and during
the time he was away, Miss Syd's care was taken over by
one of the professor's younger colleagues. When the young
doctor reviewed her chart, he was appalled to learn that
Miss Syd was being treated with medicines that were many
decades out of date. Didn't the professor know that there
were much better medicines for treating her blood pressure

and heart failure? So the young doctor would need to radically change this woman's medical regimen.

"Ms. Blasingame," the doctor greeted his new patient on their first meeting.

"Miss Syd," she corrected him, not too pleased with this substitute doctor who looked young enough to be her great-grandchild.

"Miss Syd," the doctor responded. "Tell me about yourself."

There ensued a long conversation with Miss Syd doing most of the talking and the doctor most of the listening. What the doctor learned was that Miss Syd was still living alone and caring for herself but had some trouble keeping things straight in her mind. She had learned to compensate for that by carefully organizing the things that were really important for her to do. For example, she knew exactly what each of the pills she was taking looked like and associated their appearance with the prescribed dose and frequency— the little white pill was once each morning, the larger oval pill was once in the morning and once at bedtime. She had this regimen down pat and it hadn't been changed in several years.

The doctor pondered Miss Syd's story. She had lived almost a century, was doing pretty well, and making certain that she took medicines right required a lot of effort on her part. Changing to the new pills he was considering would not be so easy for her. They looked different than the pills she had been taking and the timing of the doses would be different. The new regimen would be a big change in Miss Syd's life and it wasn't certain, even if she managed to take the pills as directed, that she would feel a lot better than she felt now. The doctor didn't change Miss Syd's medicines and she continued to do well. The rules would have said to change her to the pills that had been shown in large controlled clinical trials to be more effective than the ones she was taking. But Miss Syd was an exception. She had her own special story.

The good doctor is a student of both the rules and the exceptions and is thoroughly aware of the difference. Like her fellow medical scientists, she values hard data, the analyzed experiences of groups of patients, but she also values anecdotes. If Portland, Oregon-based infectious disease specialist and science-based medicine advocate Mark Crislip really believes, as he has said, that the three most dangerous words in a doctor's vocabulary are "in my experience," one wonders how he would go about dealing with the health care of a unique human being, like you.

It is certainly true that the practitioner who bases general use of an intervention on experiences with a couple of patients (anecdote) rather than the results of controlled trials (data) is skating on very thin ice. Even though we know that, since we (both doctors and patients) are human, we still tend to be easy marks for a good story. In fact, if our brains hadn't evolved in that direction, our species might not have survived so long. Anecdotes about the location of food or mortal danger must have given some early humans an advantage, and the risk of not believing those stories when they were true (false negatives) would have been greater than the risk of believing them when they were not true (false positives). Maybe that did something to how our brains decide what to believe. For whatever reason, it does seem as though there is something about stories which captivates us.

Although scientists are human and, like everyone else, naturally inclined to believe anecdotes, they try hard to resist that inclination. For example, the common erroneous conclusion that event A causes event B because B is sometimes seen to follow A, especially as exploited by public figure testimonials, drives a thinking doctor crazy. We mentioned earlier the claim that vaccination causes autism, and that is a prime example of how this fallacy can be used by public figures to perpetuate a falsehood that a lot of people find attractive regardless of the science. As absurd as it seems, anecdote sometimes trumps data and the consequences are not always good. Before you let your evolutionary history get the better of your logic, you need to remember how bailing water from the sea is associated with the ebbing tide.

Scientists in general are very hard on anecdotal evidence. They claim it is not based on facts; unscientific; often no more than a casual observation; and commonly just undocumented rumor. But the good doctor, even in this age of digitization, still sees value in carefully considered anecdotes, both those that she encounters first-hand and the ones that appear in the medical literature as *case reports*.

Case reports are accounts of singular or rare clinical events that are thoroughly documented by qualified professionals. They are unusual things that actually happened and they are valuable because they document things that *can* happen, no matter how rarely. They are the exceptions, which is why they are so interesting. Sure, they're interesting because unusual things always are, but they are also important because there is a chance, no matter how remote, that you might be an exception. Your doctor (assuming she is a good sort) never forgets that. She is an avid reader of case reports and enters them, with care, into the body of information that she uses to make clinical decisions. This doctor couldn't be happier if you behave exactly as the population data predicts, but she is always alert to the possibility that you may not.

After all, even a single event, an anecdote, is information, whether it's typical of a larger group of observations or is one of a kind. If something is observed to happen only once, that doesn't mean it didn't happen, nor does it mean that it won't ever happen again. Statisticians hate the single observation, the $N=1$, because they have no way to deal with it. They even have a device, Chauvenet's criterion, for getting rid of those pesky outliers. But each of us *is* an N of 1 and there is always the possibility that we will turn out to be unlike most of our kind, an outlier, sooner or later. The good doctor plays by the rules when they work, but she is also ready to deal with the exceptions because she sees them every day as she goes about caring for real human beings with real problems.

And this doctor is fascinated by your personal story. Remember Osler's admonition, "Listen to the patient, he is telling you the diagnosis." Patients' stories of their illnesses have been the essence of medical care from the time of Hippocrates and probably earlier. Although they could do a lot of harm (bloodletting, leeches, etc.), about the only constructive thing a doctor could do for much of history was to listen and try to understand disease in the context of the individual person who suffered from it. But as the science of health gained credibility and prominence, the role of narrative in health care ebbed. Emphasis on a structured approach to evidence-based care and increasing demands for doctor efficiency threatened the art of the medical narrative—even of an adequate history—with total extinction.

A lot of doctors in the trenches protested that this evidence-based thing often didn't make complete sense when facing a real person with a real, immediate problem. The generalizations didn't always fit the situation—the studies were done in different kinds of people, or the patient at hand had several complicating factors not dealt with by the evidence. These guys on the front lines know anecdotes; they face a clinic full of them every day. The term "personalized medicine" arose and numerous apologias appeared attempting with some success to reconcile the two approaches. They are after all complementary if, and only if, one's response to the marshalled evidence is something like, "well maybe, let's see how it fits with my patient in exam room four."

This recognition that who you are is inseparable from your medical condition has led to a resurgence of emphasis on the personal story as a critical component of care—*narrative-based medicine*. This is more than personalized medicine as the term is commonly used, more than even the intricate details of your biology. The most sophisticated wearable sensors won't capture this. You will not find in your genome, even when it is completely sequenced, the complete story of how interactions between you, your illness, your life experiences, and your doctor affect how well you do. In *How Doctors Think*, Katherine Montgomery, professor of medical humanities at Northwestern University, writes, "The interpretive reasoning required to understand symptoms and signs and to reach a diagnosis is represented in all its situated and circumstantial uncertainty in narrative." As Amy McGuire says, "There is no genome for the human spirit."

But the medical narrative is not just the patient's story. There is a rich history of elegant narrative inspired by clinical medicine (think Chekhov, William Carlos Williams) that brings insight into how humans deal with infirmity. The good doctor has read a lot of that literature and other classical narratives of the human condition, and it influences how she perceives you, your illness, and her own place in that complex circumstance. There may be competent doctors who are not familiar with the fecund literary history of the profession, but such doctors are missing something important that can affect how well patients do. There is some evidence that including appreciation of medicine's literary history in doctors' training can cause "significant improvements in . . . patients' health and quality of life." The point is elegantly made by David Watts in his article in *Perspective*, "Cure for the Common Cold." "Hippocrates said," Watts writes, "that some patients get well only by the goodness of their physicians." And further, "Imaginative literature shows the richness of human relationships not by trying to direct our thinking, as didactic lectures do, but by inviting us to experience lives outside our own." The good doctor knows that and searches in that literature for those embedded clues "that teach us how to live with grace in a difficult world." That's a large part of the reason why she is the good doctor.

Your doctor also has a personal story. She is well aware of what she brings to this relationship and pays attention to how her story might affect what goes on between the two of you. After all, the doctor has her own repertoire of biases, beliefs, attitudes, experiences, principles, and needs that can affect how your story registers and can threaten her objectivity if she isn't careful. Knowing that, this doctor takes the time and energy to reflect on the meaning and implications of her experiences; that's how she continues to learn about the humanity of disease.

Your doctor may well have dealt with a serious illness of her own—experienced health care from the other side. That experience can seriously affect how a doctor practices medicine. It can awaken empathy, awareness of small things that affect a patient but that easily go unnoticed by one who hasn't been there. The feelings that a doctor has when faced with a serious health problem can be surprising.

Alfred S. Reinhart was a Harvard medical student in the 1930s when he developed subacute bacterial endocarditis, an infection on a rheumatic heart valve that at the time was uniformly fatal. He was cared for by the legendary physician Soma Weiss, who observed, "the emotional reaction of A.S.R. . . . was not fundamentally different from that of any other person suffering from a hopeless disease." Sick doctors are, foremost, sick people. But the view from the other side, a personal experience with illness, can change how a doctor goes about caring for others. A close encounter with the real possibility of dying brings a new perspective that can refine a doctor's sense of empathy for sick patients. Upon being told that he had prostate cancer, a physician friend wrote the following:

"This is harder than I thought it would be. It is not a surprise. My father died of prostate cancer when I was fifteen.

The disease is no stranger. My PSA has been on the rise for over a year. The damn thing was there . . . so this is not a surprise. But that doesn't matter, doesn't soften the blow of finality, irrevocability. I have cancer. I am not the same person I was fifteen minutes ago, before I had cancer."

Our friend was not the same doctor after dealing with his own serious illness. He was a better one.

Although science dominates a doctor's education, doctors of medicine are different from scientists because they treat patients. The good doctor understands a lot about how science advances and values the results of rigorously done experiments. But she is not a human body mechanic; such a job would never have attracted her. This doctor considers herself a healer, a curer of physical disease, sure, but considerably more than that. She has tried hard to prepare herself for confronting what pediatric neurologist Philip Overby describes as "the human encounter with the sick and desperate, the brave and dying, the healed and grateful."

This doctor learned somewhere along the way, probably not in medical school, to pay a lot of attention to narratives from history and literature, and to reflect often and intensely on the meaning of her own story. But she knows above all that the most important narrative in this relationship we call clinical medicine is yours. She hasn't just read *The Care of the Patient*, Francis Peabody's classic 1927 lecture to Harvard medical students, she really believes that "The good physician knows his patients through and through, and his knowledge is bought dearly. Time, sympathy and understanding must be lavishly dispensed." She listens.

She listens for the same reason that William Osler listened, to let you tell her the diagnosis. What in medical records is labeled *history of the present illness* is a detailed account of your symptoms arranged into a chronology of your illness. The doctor then compares the content and pattern of your symptoms to the many templates of known diseases, searching for the best fit. The history will suggest what tests might help confirm the diagnosis. It's important to get the story straight if you want to get to the right diagnosis.

But that is only part of the reason for you to tell your story. This is where your doctor gets to know who you are. Your story is not just your symptoms arranged in time but how you responded to the symptoms . . . Worried? Afraid? Confused? Terrified? And how did the people around you— family, friends, colleagues—respond? Did your symptoms remind you of previous experiences of either yourself or a loved one and if so how did those turn out? What about this illness interferes with the things you treasure most in life? This is a conversation between you and your doctor meant to make you as comfortable as possible revealing everything about yourself that might affect the course of your illness or influence the direction of your treatment. It will probably take more than fifteen minutes.

So telling your story is both the path to a diagnosis and a conversation that lays the foundation of a doctor-patient relationship that will be invaluable as you and your doctor plan what to do and go about doing it. But there is more to it. There is pretty good evidence that just telling your story can make you healthier.

Writing about prior traumatic experiences boosted the immune response of a group of New Zealand medical students to hepatitis vaccination. When they were asked to write about their stressful experiences, people with asthma had improved lung function, and people with arthritis had decreased disease activity. So your doctor listens to your story not only because it is essential for getting to the right diagnosis, helps establish the all-important doctor-patient relationship, and influences a course of therapy, but also because she also knows that narrative-based medicine may have some direct fringe benefits.

Doctors who read this will say sure, it's easy for you guys to talk about lavishly dispensing time, sympathy, and understanding, but you don't have a practice manager breathing down your neck, and you're ignoring how lavishly one must bestow time on the electronic medical record. There just isn't time in an active practice today to do this sort of thing.

A doctor with appropriate skills may not need to spend all that much time with you to get the job done. A 2002 *British Medical Journal* report says that less than one percent of patients of physicians trained in *active listening* needed more than five minutes of spontaneous talking time. So the thinking doctor has learned the necessary skills to practice narrative-based medicine and tries to be as efficient as she can be doing it, but she takes whatever time is needed because she believes Francis Peabody's claim that it is "that personal bond which forms the greatest satisfaction of the practice of medicine." That's why she wanted to be a doctor in the first place, and she tries hard to remember that in spite of pressures that try to push her in another direction.

The electronic health record (EHR) has turned out to be one of those pressures. The EHR was supposed to give your doctor more time to be the kind of doctor she tries to be, but although it has some positives, in its present form it is a time and effort sink that can make her job harder.

It wasn't supposed to be that way and the EHR has done some good things—brought some organization to the medical record and detected some errors in ordered treatments. But that has been at the price of pulling the doctor away from the people she ought to be spending time with. In the *Journal of the American Medical Association*, Jayshil Patel writes that since using the electronic record in one hospital, the medical house staff spend twelve percent of their day with patients and forty percent of their time in front of a computer.

In many clinic exam rooms, the center of attention has shifted from the patient to a computer keyboard and screen mounted on a mobile base that trails the doctor around like a trained puppy. So far, the good doctor has resisted admitting a computer into her exam room; she is jealous of that sacred space reserved for her and her patient. But she pays a big price for that choice. She has to spend a lot of her own time entering all of her patients' information into the database. She can't bill for that and it surely doesn't do much for the quality of her private life. It is no surprise that the price is just more than many doctors are willing to pay.

Solutions have been tried, including the use of a scribe to enter the data while the doctor sees the patient. So now the sacred exam room space is violated with not only an ugly machine but also with a stranger who has nothing to do with what is happening except to record it; not ideal would be a serious understatement. If the enormous potential of the

EHR and other computer-related enhancements of medical practice is to be realized, it will be necessary to do some serious rethinking of the whole approach.

A contemplative doctor is well aware of the difference between the rule (evidence) and the exception (anecdote) and values them both in making decisions about your personal care. Canadian communications expert Jilleen Kosko and her colleagues at the University of Alberta ask whether (to paraphrase the title of their paper) *evidence-based medicine and the anecdote are uneasy bedfellows or an ideal couple?* They can probably be either depending on the situation and the people involved, but both are critical to the practice of good medicine. The relationship between evidence-based and narrative-based medicine may have some rocky times but this is not likely to be a short term affair.

Your personal story is critical to your health care. The doctor doesn't tell you what is wrong or right with you, you tell the doctor that. If your doctor is good at what she does, she listens. She listens very carefully. So you best pay attention to yourself. You'd better be in touch with who you are and what you are feeling, get your story straight. Most likely your health care will never be any better than your story.

Anecdotes can be what connect you to the data. That connection needs to be made although sometimes it may be too tenuous to be of much use. What if you're a Black Swan? Well, that's up to you and your doctor to figure out.

CHAPTER 13

An Expert Escort from Guidelines to Protocols

Guideline: *a thing that helps someone to form an opinion
or make a decision or calculation*
Protocol: *a detailed plan of a scientific or medical
experiment, treatment, or procedure*
—Merriam Webster Dictionary

Colin (not his real name), a thirty-seven-year-old-man, was admitted to the hospital with stomach pain, headache, vomiting, back pain, and fever. Two hours earlier, he had taken a dose of antibiotic prescribed by his dentist for a tooth infection, but he was a healthy guy, in good physical shape, and not taking any medicines regularly. He was obviously very sick when he arrived at the hospital. He was sweaty, his blood pressure was on the low side, and he had a fever and a rash on his back. His heart was racing, he was breathing too fast, and his fingers were blue. Intravenous fluids didn't help much and he was transferred to the intensive care unit. His clinical picture looked exactly like sepsis, a blood stream infection with bacteria that is often fatal, although it wasn't at all clear why he should have such a disorder. There is a rational formula for choosing what antibiotics to give a patient with this diagnosis while trying to identify the specific offending germ, and Colin was started on the four drugs recommended by those guidelines. Over the next two days Colin's liver and kidneys started failing and his blood cell counts started showing an increase in the number of eosinophils, a specific kind of white cell not usually associated with sepsis. Colin's doctors, alert to the possibility that their diagnosis might be wrong in spite of his classic signs and symptoms, concluded that he didn't have sepsis at all, but was suffering from drug reaction eosinophilia with systemic symptoms (DRESS) syndrome, a disorder that was made worse by antibiotics. All antibiotics were discontinued and Colin eventually left the hospital with everything back to normal, a very fortunate beneficiary of a successful navigation of the bridge of maybes from population based evidence to personalized treatment.

"Why the eosinophilia?" his doctors must have thought as they were treating what looked exactly like a straightforward case of sepsis with drugs that were killing their patient. But, sepsis doesn't cause eosinophilia. Well, maybe in this particular case it's something else, even though it looks for all the world like sepsis . . . except for those pesky eosinophils. Had his doctors ignored or failed to notice this inconsistency in the data and continued the antibiotics, Colin would have died. His doctors would have rationalized that sepsis is often fatal even with the best possible treatment. The lesson is that even the most carefully developed guidelines may not prescribe the best protocol for a specific case. Colin was fortunate to have doctors who never stopped looking for clues that what they were doing was wrong—pondering the maybes. That saved Colin's life.

Richard Parker (a physiologist friend, not the *Life of Pi* tiger) is fond of this joke: A general and his lieutenant are standing together viewing the battlefield. They have suffered major losses and are reduced to only a few ragtag troops. On the horizon are hundreds of enemy troops advancing rapidly toward their position. Panic in his voice, the lieutenant asks, "What should we do, general?" The general, his tone supremely confident, replies, "Lieutenant, I suggest we surround them and attack from all sides." Exasperated, the lieutenant responds, "We have only a handful of exhausted and injured men, general, how do you propose we do that?" "Strategy," replies the general, "is my job; tactics is yours." Maybe there is a rough analogy in the relationship between guidelines and protocols in medicine—the experts do strategy (guidelines), the tactics (protocols) are up to you and your doctor.

The very fact that the terms *guideline* and *protocol* are often confused may be a symptom of a potentially serious problem. A guideline without conditions, i.e., absent the maybes, becomes a protocol, and that can be a fatal error. Guidelines are what you get from expert analyses of all of the available evidence from studies in groups of people, but they should not *dictate* the details of treatment of an individual person. Guidelines are generalities. They don't write prescriptions or doctors' orders. When you are ill, what you need is a protocol. Getting from a guideline to a protocol is getting from evidence-based to personalized medicine. The only path that connects the two is a bridge of maybes. Take the maybe out of guideline and the bridge is burned; your doctor is no longer treating you.

Does it have to be that way? Why isn't it possible to write guidelines with no question marks that apply to everybody, no questions asked? After all, this isn't rocket science! Well, that's right, it's not rocket science, it's a lot more complicated than that. The good doctor knows something about how guidelines come about, and she's not about to use them as protocols to treat you without seriously questioning whether they are the best she can do for you in your specific situation.

Here are some things that this doctor knows about guidelines. As is said of success, practice guidelines have many fathers. That is, they are generated separately by several different groups, each with their own interests: the federal government (see the National Guideline Clearinghouse); a host of medical societies; the Cochrane Collaboration; entities that pay the medical bills; and various health care systems. Guidelines are influenced by the opinions and clinical experience of the *experts* chosen by the sponsoring organizations to write them. If the organizations are doing their job, they choose *experts* who are friendly to their special interests. There are a lot of special interests—controlling costs, protecting turf, favoring constituents (like doctors, risk managers, or politicians), maximizing reimbursement, etc.—that are not necessarily focused primarily on what is best for you. And then because of unconscious bias, other misinterpretations, or absent or misleading evidence, guidelines can be just plain wrong, eventually orphaned by their failure to pass muster in the real world, but leaving some damage in their wake.

Guidelines should be flexible enough to accommodate the idiosyncrasies of specific patients, but that doesn't mean that guidelines shouldn't be taken seriously. The good doctor knows that she can't just close her eyes and do whatever the guidelines say, but she also knows that she ignores well-reasoned guidelines at her and her patients' peril.

For example, guidelines from the Cochrane Collaboration, the American Pain Society, the American Society of Interventional Pain Physicians, and the American Academy of Neurology all conclude that there is no evidence that injecting steroids into the spine results in prolonged relief of low back pain. (The Cochrane review adds the caveat that "it cannot be ruled out that specific subgroups of patients may respond to a specific type of injection therapy." Maybe it works in the "right patient.")

Spinal injection of steroids is not approved by the Federal Drug Administration for low back pain. That is what is called an off-label (the drug is approved for some diseases but not this one) use of a potent steroid, methylprednisolone. In spite of the guidelines and the lack of FDA approval, nine million times every year in this country, a steroid is injected into someone's spine to treat the incredibly common symptom of back pain. Some of those patients no doubt fit into one of the *specific subgroups likely to respond to a specific type of injection therapy*, but many do not. And there are always risks, some of which may be unsuspected even by the most alert and up-to-date doctor.

An infectious disease specialist had been puzzling over her patient with meningitis for two weeks. The patient wasn't responding to antibiotics that should have taken care of the usual causes of the disease, and no bad bugs were growing from his body fluids that were sent to the laboratory. That is until one September day when the laboratory called with the answer. Finally, a fungus was growing from the patient's spinal fluid. He had a rare and often fatal form of fungal meningitis. In response to detailed questioning about his health practices, the doctor discovered that her patient had recently had an injection of steroids into his spine to treat his chronic back pain. The source of the deadly fungus in his spinal fluid was finally traced to contaminated batches of the injected steroid solution that led to a major epidemic.

The contaminated steroid story demonstrates that the consequences of ignoring guidelines aren't just abstract medical mistakes; they can include the kinds of personal tragedies in real people that haunt a concerned doctor. Cynthia Scribe's (not her real name) friends described her as "hilarious, beautiful, and full of life." She was the primary caregiver for her husband, who was confined to a wheelchair with Lou Gehrig's disease. She lost her job and wanted to get her back pain treated while she was still covered by health insurance. A few hours after her third injection of the tainted steroid, she developed headaches. Her course was rapidly downhill and finally, after suffering several strokes, she died in a hospice surrounded by her husband and friends.

The contaminated steroids were produced by New England Compounding Center in Massachusetts, the primary supplier of the drug (methylprednisolone acetate) intended for this use. The meningitis epidemic spread to nineteen states and 720 victims, 48 of whom died. The risk of something like this is no doubt low, but also most of the patients who got the drug were unlikely to benefit from it. There are always risks, some of which can't be anticipated. The good doctor takes the Hippocratic dictum "first do no harm" seriously. If she isn't pretty sure she can help you, she'll at least do her best not to make you any worse.

So ignoring guidelines is risky even though the experts who develop them deliberately leave room for adapting the therapy to you; you could be one in a *subgroup that is likely to respond* in spite of a negative guideline recommendation. A thinking doctor understands how important uncertainties in the guidelines are in making your treatment personal, but she doesn't take the uncertainties as a license to freelance. She won't advise you to have a therapy based solely on her limited experience if that differs radically from the larger body of evidence. This doctor has vivid memories of her patients. She cherishes those memories, and, though they do not trump the evidence, they may help as the two of you ponder difficult options. A single experience is a dangerous basis for deciding on a treatment, but experience can be a valuable aid as you and your doctor wend your way over the bridge from guidelines to protocols.

So, your doctor generates a protocol that is especially yours, but it may not be unique in the strict sense. Here is an oversimplified example that illustrates the point. Patients with cystic fibrosis (CF), a genetic disease that mostly affects the lungs, often have spells where their lung infection takes over and they have to be treated in the hospital. There is a lot of evidence that several interventions are effective—intravenous antibiotics, chest physiotherapy, inhaled medications, etc. So, based on guidelines carefully developed from the available evidence, CF doctors usually have "protocols" that include each of the evidence-based interventions. These show up automatically on the doctor's orders in the admission part of the electronic medical record. But, isn't that just rote adherence to the guidelines? No, it's not, because there are options. Choice of antibiotics will depend on what bacteria are growing out of the lungs and whether the patient is allergic to anything. Frequency and dose of inhaled medications will depend on the patient's size, ability to cooperate, how they have responded to such treatments in the past, and many other variables that are unique to a specific situation. The point is that your specific treatment comes from a careful distillation of the evidence, your idiosyncrasies, and your doctor's and others' experience. And your doctor doesn't just design your protocol and go home. She pays continual attention to how you are responding, ever alert to the possibility that you could be an outlier and that your protocol might need revising at any time.

As she does her best to give you the best medical care possible, the good doctor is always aware of how important it is to recognize the difference between guidelines and protocols. Statistical data from population studies are invaluable, and the more there is of such evidence, the better. But *evidence-based medicine* done right uses evidence to inform care related decisions rather than as a precise prescription for what to do for an individual patient.

When deciding what to do to be as healthy as you can be or to treat your disease when you get sick, you want the best possible chance to do what is best for you. That means clearly understanding the difference between guidelines and protocols, a distinction that you can't reliably make on your own. Far and away your best resource is a thinking doctor who listens well, knows you, and knows what she is doing—a doctor whom you trust, and with whom you've built a relationship that is as equal a partnership as possible.

The internet doesn't do a very good job of even getting the facts straight and pretty much misses entirely the nuanced distinction between guidelines and protocols. If you ever feel inclined to blindly trust what you get from the public media, the independent website http://HealthNewsReview. org ought to give you pause; they critique news stories about medical claims. They reviewed around 1,800 stories from a dozen or more reputable organizations in the U.S. and found that seventy percent didn't accurately report cost, potential for benefit, and potential for harm. And these were stories from reputable sources. Imagine the reliability of unfiltered information from infomercials, public personalities, and the like.

"Your health is your most valuable asset" is more than a shopworn phrase, it is an essential fact of life. If you don't believe that now, you will as soon as you have to deal with a serious disease; there is nothing like being really sick to rearrange one's priorities. We are fortunate to live in a free country where a lot of resources are available that can help us to be as healthy as we can be. But the freedom that gives us access to good information also opens the door to misinformation that can lead us in the wrong direction. You and your doctor need to work together to parse the facts and fictions to your advantage. You need the knowing doctor's steady hand if you're to make it safely across the bridge of maybes.

You would be foolish to go it alone. You'll have gut reactions, but don't trust them. Viscera have their critical functions, but they are unreliable discerners of truth.

CHAPTER 14

The Benefits of Ignorance

Real knowledge is to know the extent of one's ignorance.
—CONFUCIUS

So this curious, constantly thinking doctor relies heavily on ignorance as she tries to figure out how the available evidence fits you personally. She is keenly aware of and intrigued by the fact that ignorance—the things nobody knows—is why we learn new things. There are always a few curious, daring, and adventurous souls who feel compelled to go off searching for the unknown answers, and sometimes what they find astounds us.

This good doctor read somewhere in her youth that "a good question is worth a lot more than a mediocre fact," and she took that dictum to heart. In fact, if her medical school teachers had a criticism of their star student, it would have been that she asked too many questions. Her common response to a pontificating professor was to ask *why*? Pontificating professors tend to be pretty satisfied with accepted dogma and don't always respond well to a too inquisitive student. But this student persisted and even now all of the stuff that is either completely unknown or at best uncertain haunts and excites her. Excites her because she knows that ignorance drives discovery and discovery is the pulsating life blood of medicine. Discovery saves lives. The good doctor loves the lore of medical discovery and she often ponders those dramatic stories.

A surgeon's dissatisfaction with what he didn't know changed a certain death sentence into a manageable disease. Leonard Thompson's family doctor knew he had diabetes and that eating sugar was bad for him, but the doctor had no idea what caused the disease or what to do to prevent the young man's premature death. A near starvation diet had kept him alive for a few years, but the fourteen-year-old was down to sixty-five pounds and drifting in and out of coma when he was admitted to the Toronto General Hospital in January of 1922. He was on his last legs. He would surely not leave the hospital alive.

But a few years earlier, Frederick Banting, a little known Toronto orthopaedic surgeon, had been driven by what neither he nor anyone knew about diabetes to convince his department chairman to grubstake his effort to see whether maybe it had something to do with the pancreas. In a series of experiments in dogs, Banting and his medical student assistant, Charles Best, showed that something produced by the pancreas (they initially called it isletin since it came from nests of pancreas cells that looked like islets under the microscope) did indeed regulate blood sugar in dogs and cured their experimental diabetes.

Leonard Thompson was selected as the first human to receive this new substance (now called insulin). The initial injection of an impure preparation helped some but also caused a severe allergic reaction. Injection of biochemist J. B. Collip's pure preparation of the substance was begun on

January 23, 1922, with stunning results. Leonard's life was saved! A medical miracle! By 1923 the Eli Lilly Company was producing massive amounts of insulin, which has saved the lives of millions of diabetics over the years. What his doctors didn't know about diabetes saved Leonard Thompson's life and the lives of millions since.

The diabetes story and others like it continue to inspire practitioners of medicine. But they aren't just history lessons. Understanding that ignorance is a powerful source of life-saving discovery keeps the inquisitive doctor on the lookout for more recent examples. She finds examples because she looks for them but also because her curious mind is open to consider even the strangest possibilities. She knows the extent of her ignorance.

Sometimes lives are saved by interventions that seem bizarre at first blush. University of Colorado surgeon Ben Eisman and his colleagues may have known in 1958 that millennia earlier, Chinese patients drank what they called "yellow soup" to treat intestinal ailments. But the Colorado group certainly did not know the cause of pseudomembranous colitis (it was later determined to be a really nasty bacterium, *Clostridium difficile*—*C. diff*), a serious disease that often didn't respond very well to antibiotics. And they didn't know what would happen if they infused fecal matter from a normal person into the lower intestine of patients with the disease. They knew, however, that their four patients, critically ill with this devastating disease, were not responding to conventional therapy and were likely to die unless they did something else. Hoping that some factor in the fecal material from a normal person would counteract whatever evil lurked in their patients' bowels, in 1958 Eisman and his colleagues performed fecal matter transplants (FMT) in their four critically ill patients and reported the results in an article titled, "Fecal enema as an adjunct in the treatment of pseudomembranous colitis" in the journal *Surgery*. The results were dramatic. All four patients recovered from their colitis, their lives saved because their doctors were driven by what they didn't know.

Cheryl Cawthon's (not her real name) doctor in Providence, Rhode Island, was near his wits end. Ms. Cawthon was a seventy-nine-year-old retired nurse. When she developed diverticulitis, an intestinal ailment resulting from infections of small outpouchings in the wall of the large bowel that occasionally occur with age, her doctor treated her with seriously strong antibiotics, the standard approach. Her diverticulitis resolved, but, as sometimes happens after treatment with potent antibiotics, Ms. Cawthon developed a persistent intestinal infection with *C. diff* that caused chronic debilitating diarrhea. Her doctor treated her now and again with a course of antibiotics, and she would get a little better for a while and then the diarrhea would return. Her doctor had no idea what to do next, but he did know that one of the faculty at a local university was doing some kind of unusual treatment and referred Ms. Cawthon there. The proposed treatment sounded strange, but also made some sense to the retired nurse. The idea was to overwhelm the pesky *C. diff* that had set up housekeeping in her bowel with a mass of bacteria that enabled the bowel to function normally, hoping the good guys would crowd out the bad guys. Which they did. Ms. Cawthon's son dutifully agreed to donate the material to be transplanted and two days after the FMT Ms. Cawthon's diarrhea disappeared, never to return. Another triumph of medical ignorance.

A randomized study published in the *New England Journal of Medicine* in 2013 reported that FMT cured 94 percent of patients with *C.diff* infections while antibiotics only cured 31 percent. FMT was so successful that the controlled study was stopped early because it was felt unethical to withhold such an effective treatment from anyone with the disease. There are some reports that FMT may be beneficial in a number of other intestinal diseases that have been resistant to therapy. What doctors don't know is the engine of discovery.

The good doctor also knows from her personal experience and from stories of how major scientific discoveries were made that, as Yogi Berra is supposed to have said, "you can see a lot just by looking." She looks intently at even the most common-place events because she knows it can pay off. She may know, for example, that biochemist Stan Cohen's careful scrutiny of something simple that he didn't expect wound up changing how we think about cancer and won him the Nobel Prize.

Since he worked with mice in his laboratory, no doubt Dr. Cohen knew that newborn mice don't open their eyes until some days after birth, but he may not have known very much about the details of what happened after birth that allowed the pups' eyes to open. Stan and Rita Levi-Montalcini, his colleague at Washington University, weren't interested in why newborn mice's eyes opened. They were focused on factors that caused nerves to grow, and mouse salivary glands were rich sources of the nerve growth factor they were studying. However, when they injected crude salivary gland preparations into mice, Cohen noticed that the newborn pups' eyelids opened ahead of schedule. A pure preparation of nerve growth factor didn't have that effect. Something in the crude preparation was causing the eyelid skin (epidermis) to grow over the edges of the lids freeing the lids to open prematurely. Hmmm, a factor that stimulates epidermis to grow, Dr. Cohen must have thought; that's interesting. He decided to find out what that factor was and published the discovery of epidermal growth factor in 1960. That discovery, based on a prescient observation of an unanticipated experimental side effect, has turned out to have major implications for cancer biology and potentially for cancer treatment. Dr. Cohen shared the 1986 Nobel Prize in Physiology or Medicine with Dr. Levi-Montalcini. Ignorance may or may not be bliss, but it is a powerful driver of discoveries that could save your life.

Columbia University neuroscientist Stuart Firestein's fascinating little book, *Ignorance: How it Drives Science,* resonates with any curious mind. Appalled at the discovery that most of his neuroscience students thought that their big textbook contained pretty much everything there was to know about the subject, Firestein began a course that he titled *Ignorance,* which became the stimulus for his book.

Conventional teaching that knowledge drives out ignorance is, Firestein says, exactly 180 degrees at odds with the truth that knowledge produces ignorance. The more we know, the more we know that we don't know. The bigger the island of knowledge, the longer the shoreline of ignorance. "The known is never safe," Firestein writes. "The more exact the fact, the less reliable it is likely to be." His description of how uncertainly science proceeds uses an unattributed proverb, "It is very difficult to find a black cat in a dark room. Especially when there is no cat." The thinking doctor often feels like she is groping around in the dark trying to locate the black cat that may not exist, and she is perfectly willing to let you to know that.

Like scientists in general, medical scientists are more excited by the unexpected than by proof of what they thought they already knew. We learn by being wrong. And medicine is very good at being wrong, which makes the field fascinating to a lot of bright and committed people. Some of those exceptional people are so taken with the uncertainties, the questions unanswered, that they dedicate their lives to efforts to discover. These are the clinician-scientists who are intrigued by the uncertainties but not satisfied with them. These are the bright and committed people who lies awake nights pondering unknowns and wondering what an unexpected result of an experiment is trying to say. The good doctor who practices medicine stays in touch with those people and will be sure that you benefit from their discoveries when the time comes.

If ignorance is such a powerful stimulus for discovery, shouldn't all doctors learn that in medical school? Perhaps they should, but too often they don't. Medical education is particularly guilty of treating ignorance as the enemy, a dark force to be frightened away by the bright light of knowledge. Somewhere along the way, medical students often become convinced that they just need to know the facts with little appreciation for how those facts cower before the vastly greater power of ignorance. The process of *training* doctors as opposed to *educating* them can stifle curiosity, the innate fascination with the unknown. Too frequently doctors complete their training with no clear grasp of how important ignorance—a pervasive sense of maybe—is when dealing with the incredible complexity of human biology.

There is some pretty convincing evidence that doctors in training aren't learning how to deal with what they don't know. Recognizing that effective clinical decisions require that the doctor "disclose personal uncertainty," Professor of Family Medicine Christy Ledford and colleagues surveyed family practice training programs to determine "How We Teach U.S. Medical Students to Negotiate Uncertainty in Clinical Care," the title of their publication in the journal *Family Medicine*. We would expect that family practice programs would do a better job of recognizing the need for teaching uncertainty than most other medical specialties. They probably do, but apparently they still don't do it very well. Most of the program directors agree that teaching skills in dealing with uncertainty is important to do, but Ledford, et al. conclude that, "over half of all clerkships are missing an opportunity . . . to help learners develop competencies related to . . . uncertainty management, such as listening attentively, having a compassionate presence, and providing patient-centered communication." Your good doctor learns this stuff on her own. Many of her peers do not.

It is not a lot of consolation when you need a doctor to find out that being wrong is an essential part of medical practice and that a lot of practitioners don't know how to deal with that. Uncertainty, that ubiquitous maybe, is always lurking in the wings so that decisions are always risky, whether or not the decision maker admits it.

Granted that there is no font of absolute certainty in medicine, how can you best stack the deck in your favor? First, you can look on the bright side of *maybe*, see possibilities as the many good ways things could turn out. There is no doubt that your attitude toward your health has a potent effect, for better or worse. But that's not enough. You also need a doctor whom you trust and who takes you on as the real person you are. But there are always risks and if you're told otherwise, you're not being dealt with honestly. So you're not looking for a doctor who claims perfection; a doctor like that is going to be wrong and may not know it. You want a doctor who knows the risks and how to minimize them. That doctor knows the extent of her ignorance. She has long since made peace with uncertainty.

CHAPTER 15

The Laying On of Hands

It is believed by experienced doctors that the heat which oozes out of
the hand, on being applied to the sick, is highly salutary.
—HIPPOCRATES, fifth century BC

The thoughtful, caring doctor will touch you with her
hands. She will do that for three reasons: to sense what's
going on inside; to connect with who you are; and because
she is a healer.

TO SENSE WHAT'S GOING ON INSIDE

Medical students take a course called *Physical Diagnosis*
which is supposed to teach them how to use their senses to
detect clues to how well a patient's vital organs are doing
their jobs. There are four parts to the physical examination:
inspection (looking carefully at the body's color, contours, and
other features that can be seen with the naked eye); *percussion*
(thumping on the chest, abdomen, etc. and registering both
the sound and the feel of the response); *palpation* (poking and
prodding all of the relevant areas to determine size, contour,
and sensitivity of the patient's internal organs); and finally
auscultation (exploring each body area with a stethoscope,

listening carefully for normal and abnormal sounds and registering which organs seem to be producing them). There
was a time when this was the most important course in the
education of an aspiring doctor.

So when you go to the doctor you can confidently expect
to be looked at, thumped on, poked, prodded, and listened
to, right? Well, you shouldn't get your hopes up. While
those things are true if you're seeing the kind of doctor we
are describing, she may be in the minority these days. After
all, now that we have x-rays, ultrasound, CAT scans, MRIs,
and all those other technologies that see what's going on
inside with considerable precision, why does the doctor need
to master an approach as low tech as the traditional physical exam? A lot of doctors just don't see the point. Famed
Harvard cardiologist Roman DeSanctis jokingly lamented,
"If you come to our hospital missing a finger, no one will
believe you until we get a CAT scan, an MRI, and an orthopedic consult. We just don't trust our senses."

And machines can only see what the doctor tells them
to look for. Depending on where they're looking and how,
even the most sophisticated technologies can miss a diagnosis that is readily made by a careful physical exam, which
has serious implications for therapy.

Physician writer Sandeep Jauhar recounts his father's
experience, which illustrates this point. Dr. Jauhar's father
was taken to the hospital because of episodes of tingling in
his left arm. Fearing a stroke, the neurologist who saw him
ordered a CT scan of his brain, which was normal, and then
an MRI of his head, which was also normal. Undaunted, the
neurologist admitted the patient to the hospital and started

him on blood thinning medicines. To be sure there wasn't a blood clot in his heart that had broken off and gone to his brain, the patient had an echocardiogram, then an ultrasound of the artery in his neck, and a battery of other expensive tests, all of which were normal. After a while his symptoms got better and he was sent home with a bunch of medicines and a return appointment with the neurologist. Three days later the symptoms came back worse than ever. He was taken back to the ER and had another normal CT scan. Finally a nurse noticed that when she had the patient turn his head a certain way, it caused the tingling in his arm exactly as he had experienced it all along. Several doctors confirmed that observation making the diagnosis of a pinched nerve in his neck that was the explanation for his discomfort. Twenty thousand dollars' worth of high-tech tests were all for naught while the carefully observed response to a simple physical maneuver nailed down the problem.

The good doctor knows from personal experience that physical findings can sometimes trump the technology. And the scans she does using only her ears, eyes, and hands are done in the privacy of an exam room without elaborate equipment. She trusts her senses but also recognizes their limitations, and so she uses all of the available technology where appropriate. But she has a hard and fast rule to always start with a careful physical examination. She might think of that as something like the *rule of the gold stethoscope*. And she might explain that to herself this way:

Learning the profession I chose is, I find, a process, not an event . . . the gift that keeps on giving as they say. Still, after all these years, I learn something every day, often from unlikely sources and when I least expect it. Experiences that seem small at the time stick with me. For example, every time I face a patient I'm reminded of the gold stethoscope, an icon etched into my brain as a symbol of the importance of a thorough physical exam. My old professor Dr. Samples was the stethoscope's owner, and I learned from him the nuts and bolts of physical diagnosis. Not just how to do it, but also the value of the exercise. "Remember this gold stethoscope," he would say, brandishing his shiny pride and joy. "Nothing you will do as a doctor is more valuable than observing, touching, and listening to your patient." I remember those sessions like they were yesterday; apparently the lesson of the gold stethoscope is with me forever.

TO CONNECT WITH WHO YOU ARE

Even if she takes the time and trouble to do a complete and thorough physical exam and discovers nothing abnormal, the good doctor will still believe that the time and effort were well spent. You and your doctor need to get to know each other if you are to figure out how best to keep you healthy or get you well when the need arises. That means you have to form a relationship. Not unlike many relationships, this one has paradoxes—it is intimate but distant, revealing but secretive, caring but pragmatic. And the *laying on of hands*, the physical interaction of the doctor and the patient, is a critical part of the process. That is not only to *see what's happening inside,* but also as a ritual that gives substance to this special doctor-patient connection.

Stanford physician and author Abraham Verghese says, "When one individual (a patient) seeks help from another individual, and confides in that other person, and then incredibly, disrobes and allows touch, that has all the trappings of a ritual . . . that is fundamental to the doctor–patient relationship." The thoughtful doctor knows something about the importance of ritual, and each time she examines one of her fellow humans, she is impressed again with how important that experience is to a health care relationship that works right. That is, after all, why she chose medicine over more exclusively intellectual career possibilities; she wanted to do something to understand people and improve their lot. That is what she still finds most satisfying about her job. And that is why you want her to lay her hands on you. These might be some of this doctor's private thoughts about rituals:

Another thing I think I've learned that I was not taught in med school is that there is more to the physical examination than discovering pathology. Patients show up in my office expecting something very concrete. They expect to sit with me and recount their medical history and then they expect to be asked to take off their clothes and to be touched by me. They expect those things because that is the drill, the ritual that is part and parcel of the patient-doctor encounter. When the ritual is done, this new patient and I are connected in a different way whether or not my exam reveals anything significant about their physical state. If it goes as it should, we've laid the groundwork for the kind of relationship that is essential if our collaboration is to help this patient to be as healthy and happy as possible.

This ritual thing is not magical, mystical, or sleight-of-hand. And, although it is ritual, it is not rote. I'm paying attention, not just going through the motions. A robot can't do this! I see no con-

flict between holding to a time-honored effective ritual and my role as a clinical scientist practicing science-based medicine. We, both me and my patient, are people and people need rituals. Rituals christen us, marry us, usher us into adulthood, escort us from this mortal world into the great beyond. Connections with other people and, for the religious, even with God—marriage ceremonies, prayer, worship services, holy communion—are made more real by ritual. So when I dare to engage with another person in a sincere and very personal effort to deal with the care of their health, I am committed to bringing the best science that I can find to the task, but I will also lay my hands on that person. And both of us will benefit.

BECAUSE SHE IS A HEALER

The good doctor wants to see your disease cured, but she also wants to see your hurt healed; she knows that they are not necessarily the same thing. Some topical antibiotic cream and a bandage will hasten healing of a child's skinned knee, but if delivered along with a hug from a loving parent it will work a lot better. And you haven't grown out of your need for human touch when you hurt, although you may have some trouble admitting that even to yourself. You don't need to admit the need for touch to a caring doctor. She senses the need and lays an empathetic hand on your shoulder or takes your hand in hers at the times when those gestures are exactly what you need. She has a box of tissues handy if your tears need drying. This doctor really does feel for you and the laying on of hands is her way of sharing your experience and helping you to bear the pain, whatever its source.

You don't have to do this alone is the message. Your doctor is there for the duration and committed to getting you back to physical health and also back to the pleasures of a happy and healthy life. She is a curer but also a healer.

The good doctor is not a shaman, magician, or faith healer. Her faith is in the scientific basis of medical practice, and science is the bedrock of what she does. She does not feel that the laying on of hands transfers to you some mystical energy that summons out the evil humors of disease and pain. But that doesn't mean that the healing effects of human touch are not real. Even if she can't explain in detail the chain of physiological and biochemical events that connect the human touch with healing, she has no trouble believing that those connections exist. There is so much about the theory and practice of medicine that is unexplained. After all, that is this doctor's reason for being and why you want her as your partner in caring for your health. She might say something like this about curing and healing:

It took me a while to realize that many times my job is not done when my patient's disease or injury is cured. There wasn't much in my formal education to clue me in to the reality that human maladies have multiple dimensions and that if I am to be the doctor I aspire to be I've got to do more than prescribe an effective antibiotic or get my patient on the right dose of heart failure medicines. Those things might cure the immediate medical problem but leave the patient unhealed. And my job is not done unless the patient is healed as well as cured. Of course, if things work perfectly, the two happen together, but I can't trust that to chance. If I don't pay attention to those other dimensions of illness, my patient and I may well win the battle but lose the war.

So now I, perhaps belatedly, consider myself a healer. I've learned, mostly by trial and error, that a healing relationship with a patient involves a lot of touching, both real physical touching and the more figurative gentle bumping together of emotional boundaries. Sincere, caring, empathetic touches of a human hand, sometimes as apparently trivial as a pat on the shoulder or a handshake, can be healing gestures. Touching can make a difference.

It takes a doctor some time and experience to realize the full potential of touch in the care of her patients. Her path to that point is littered with people who were cured but not healed or who, if healed, did it without her help. The good doctor often thinks about what she could have done or been for those patients but didn't or wasn't for lack of understanding . . . or time. Time still threatens her role as healer.

Writer Malcolm Gladwell says, "What doctors and patients need is more time, not more technology." But why must it be one or the other? There is an array of powerful technologies and many more to come that will expand a doctor's access to information, her ability to measure critical structures and functions of the human body, and her capacity to make sense of it all in the unique context of you. If the interface of humans and machines works as it should, won't that give your doctor and you more face time as well as the other benefits of the technology?

Efforts to delegate health care *completely* to gadgets and computers imply a kind of assembly line medicine with homogenized care and rigid time commitments. Those may be useful tools for management, but they do not work in medical practice because every single patient a doctor sees is different. Humans are not produced on an assembly line! Health care at its most effective is a collaborative effort between you and your doctor, and it requires a special relationship between those two real people. That kind of relationship takes time and attention . . . and the laying on of hands.

PART V

Fears and Hopes for
the New Medicine

CHAPTER 16

The Fear of a Tyranny of Experts and Sensors

I worry that we could become tyrannized by a combination of experts
and sensors that have no close relationship to our priorities . . . I think
it's about this deeper connection we all have to something important.

—ATUL GAWANDE

A tyranny of experts?

There are two groups of experts who, for different reasons,
might be seen as threats to the whole health care system:
medical experts and *experts in the business of medicine*.

MEDICAL EXPERTS

The good doctor bases her decisions about your care on
evidence based guidelines developed by the experts as they
apply to you. However, she knows that occasionally those
guidelines morph, even in well-intended systems, into rigid
protocols with unintended consequences; she stays alert to
those exceptions.

Here's an example. In a hospital where a certain general
surgeon practiced, the evidence based guideline that antibiotics given intravenously to prevent infection around the
time of surgery (prophylaxis) should be begun within an

hour of the operation and discontinued twenty-four hours after the procedure was written into the standard orders as a quality assurance protocol. This surgeon had a patient with acute inflammation of the gallbladder show up at the hospital at 2:00 a.m. The doctor admitted the patient and gave admission orders that included beginning intravenous antibiotics immediately. The antibiotics were meant to treat an infection that was likely already present—therapy, not prophylaxis. The next morning, the surgeon got the patient on the OR schedule and the nurse asked if he wanted to start antibiotics before surgery. When he replied that the patient had been receiving antibiotics for the past eight hours, since being admitted, the nurse shook her head and said no, that the night nurse had delayed starting the antibiotics until within an hour of surgery, like the quality assurance protocol said. Bad medicine. Embedding decisions dictated by the experts' evidence-based guidelines into the system as a protocol that can take an important decision out of the hands of the responsible doctors risks a practice that the experts never intended. "A foolish consistency," Ralph Waldo Emerson wrote, "is the hobgoblin of little minds." Thinking people, including the good doctor, are rather fond of Mr. Emerson.

At least since early in the twentieth century, most doctors practicing in the United States have tried to base their care of patients on the best available evidence. Up until the last thirty plus years, each physician was responsible for digging up whatever evidence he or she could find, blending that with his or her personal experience and deciding for a specific patient how to proceed. As one would guess, this resulted in widely disparate practices, depending on how vigorously the doctor dug for the evidence and how the evidence was interpreted in the context of a doctor's clinical experience and the patient at hand.

Recognizing this disparity and believing that a broader and more rigorous analysis of evidence and its implications made widely available would improve care, a formal program of evidence-based medicine began in the 1960s, and evolved over the following three decades. The fully developed program has a lot of structure. There are specific rules for valuing evidence. The available evidence weighted for its scientific rigor is then used by experts to develop practice guidelines. Whole organizations spend their time searching the literature and generating documents that guide doctors in what to do in many clinical situations. The National Guideline Clearinghouse maintains a database of guidelines meant to influence practice in the clinic. That database addresses well over a thousand specific clinical situations.

Complaining about the habitual tendency of his economic advisors to equivocate (*on the one hand . . . but then on the other . . .*), President Harry Truman longed for a one-handed economist. Does evidence-based medicine threaten to neutralize our good doctor by amputating the other hand, creating an illusion of certainty that the facts don't support and so minimizing the role of the doctor's clinical judgment? There are some people who think so; evidenced based medicine has been maligned as "inconsistent with modern science, theoretically unsound, impractical and erroneous in its application," "a simplistic cookbook approach, an excuse for not thinking" that contributes to "the debasement of physicians as 'providers.'"

The good doctor knows better than that. She does not confuse evidence-based guidelines with inflexible instructions for how to take care of you; she is thoroughly aware of and comfortable with the uncertainties. But she always starts with the available evidence.

How about the teaching of medicine? Do the medical experts threaten to "tyrannize" the process of training doctors? Evidence based medicine is the touchstone of much of current medical education. Round on any ward in an academic medical center on any day and you are virtually certain to hear the term more than once. Does that mean that the intellectual part of medicine is on the road to complete automation, needing doctors only to operate the computer, recite the edicts of the experts, and write prescriptions?

The good doctor knew better than that even when she was a medical student, and her experience practicing medicine continues to impress her with the need to deal with human ambiguity as she goes about trying to translate the available evidence into actual care of real people. She was fortunate to have teachers and role models during her long period of education and training who not only knew what they were doing and why but also cared deeply for the human beings for whom they were doing it. She learned some things from those teachers.

Does our good doctor practice evidence-based medicine? She surely does, but the way she does it won't please anyone looking to eliminate the ambiguities. She pays close attention to the numbers, but she isn't driven by them; she doesn't practice exclusively digital medicine. She has great respect for science carefully done and properly interpreted, but, like Atul Gawande, the good doctor knows "that nothing is ever completely settled, that all knowledge is just probable knowledge." She knows that medical conclusions, even at their most solid, are often inexact and so she doesn't always strictly toe the "experts'" line. This doctor is okay with ambiguity and that figures into her decisions. Her brand of evidence-based medicine requires not only knowing but understanding the evidence in the full context of what is and what is not known and in the specific context of you as a unique person. She is not the experts' doctor. She is *your* doctor! If you fit with what the experts predict, that is just fine. If you don't, then "experts" be damned!

EXPERTS IN THE BUSINESS OF MEDICINE

So our good doctor will not succumb to a tyranny of the experts who compile the evidence and write the guidelines. But how about the other experts who deal with the business side of things? The evolution of American medicine into a major industry and a powerful economic engine brought with it a bevy of non-medical experts—managers, economists, efficiency experts, systems designers, etc.—who aim to structure a doctor's practice and manage her function with an eagle eye fixed on her margin, the bottom line, how much money she brings in above the total cost of her practice. Health care becomes a product, not unlike an industry-manufactured widget, and practices that work to maximize profit in the widget business are expected to do the same for the practice of medicine. This approach is what brought us, among other requirements that are unrelated to the needs of the patient, the fifteen minute office visit. Need to increase doctor efficiency, the experts asked? That's simple, just speed up the assembly line. Have the doc see more patients per unit time (which obviously means less time per patient).

Well, that approach is not working very well now, and it never will. Health care is not a product, at least not in any sense that resembles a widget. What really drives a thoughtful caring doctor to work harder and do a better job is not how much money she can generate, but how much healthier and happier she can make her patients. This brand of medicine has at its root a personal relationship between you and her. You do not go to see her to buy a product but to experience the complex processes of curing and healing that can only happen when the very best science infuses the genuine care of you as a human being. While financial incentives can change many doctors' behaviors to the detriment of their patients in the short run, there are easier ways for smart people to make money. Greed doesn't blend well with the motives that attract most bright people into a medical career. A margin-driven style of health care will not make you heathier and will have little lasting appeal to a dedicated doctor. The good doctor will not forever endure a tyranny of the business experts.

A TYRANNY OF SENSORS?

Sensors are devices that measure things and their readout is in numbers; they are the fundamental tools of digital medicine. The digitizers are convinced that if they can get enough things about you sensed and recorded numerically, they will know all they need to know to treat you as precisely as the state of medical knowledge permits; just follow the numbers. If we buy that idea, then we ought to be about capitalizing on the enormous potential of modern technology to make as many sensors as possible and to make them portable, cheap, and accurate enough to become integral to our everyday life. That is exactly what is in the works, in some cases on a rather grand scale.

Would you believe *Moonshot Medicine*? Astro Teller (although it seems unlikely, we assume that is his real name) likes that idea. Teller, grandson of Manhattan Project physicist Edward Teller, is "the captain of moonshots" at Google-X (or whatever Alphabet, Inc. decides to call it now), the innovation laboratory that brought us the eyeglass computer, the delivery drone, and the internet-beaming high altitude balloon. I mean, how hard can this medical thing be? So, Google-X is taking on a new moonshot project, the human body. They'll collect every morsel of information that there are sensors of any kind to measure from 175 normal people and use the frightening power of their computers to create a definition of health that will be a basis for detecting the earliest evidence of *unhealth* (our term) and nipping it in the bud. These guys really are thinking innovation.

The National Institutes of Health are also getting in on the act. The Institutes intend to convince one million Americans to wear some sensors of blood pressure, exercise, and other health related information that will be fed to a central repository. The information will form a database that will be bigger and more complete than anything that exists now. And, we presume, as the number of personal remote sensors, many of them wearable, proliferates to include measurements of a lot of blood chemicals, DNA sequences, and even environmental conditions and social interactions, the database will expand enormously. Imagine all of those things being sensed and recorded all day, every day, ad infinitum. Anticipating such a possibility, San Diego professor and book author Eric Topol writes that the creative destruction of medicine "is ready to go . . . because for the first time in history we can digitize humans." Our good doctor hyperventilates just thinking about it. This could redefine how she thinks about disease in general, but what gets her so excited is that it could also define your unique biology more precisely than she could have imagined. It could make your doctor a better doctor! You could be healthier! It might even save your life!

But wait. Is our usually cautious and thoughtful doctor about to succumb to the tyranny of the sensors? We hope not. More information doesn't necessarily result in better health care; it depends on how the information is understood and used. Surely the good doctor knows that, and once she comes down from her technological high she will remember the critical value of context. She may even remember a story like this one.

A seventy-five-year-old physician we know was in excellent health. He saw his internist twice a year and his physical exam, cardiogram, and blood tests were always normal. He took his daily dose of Lipitor, which dealt effectively with a high cholesterol. His diet was healthy, he kept his weight down, exercised every day, had an excellent relationship with his wife of many years, and lived a happy and interesting life. He started noticing that the detector on his treadmill occasionally failed to register his pulse rate. He was pretty sure that he had a pulse, so he felt for it. He found that when the machine didn't detect it, his pulse was irregular; most of the time it was completely normal. He had absolutely no symptoms—no pain, no palpitations, nothing. His heart rate had always been normal when he went for his regular medical checkups. He told his doctor about this occasional pulse irregularity on a routine visit and, although our friend's pulse was regular at the time, his doctor ordered an exercise test. Sure enough, at maximum exercise, his cardiogram showed a period of atrial fibrillation, a fairly common form of irregular heartbeat in a man his age. If this irregular heartbeat is constant, there all the time, it can increase the risk of stroke. But in this patient it was documented to be intermittent, which is not an emergency. However, what the cardiologist on call saw was a seventy-five year old man with atrial fibrillation. He couldn't believe that this guy had no symptoms. In fact, the cardiologist was heard dictating in his note that "the patient experienced palpitations"; he just couldn't help himself. Our friend didn't correct him; he had told the guy otherwise already.

After discussions with several doctors, the cardiologist decided that this irregular heartbeat had to be fixed. He prescribed two pills for the patient to take when he returned home. Those two pills should do the trick. Our friend took the pills, which dropped his blood pressure to frightening levels and caused him to pass out in the middle of a restaurant near his home. He was loaded into an ambulance, had yet another cardiogram, an intravenous line was started, he was given oxygen, and he was delivered to a local emergency room. He had still another cardiogram which showed that his heartbeat was now normal (as it had been when he first went for his regular checkup, before the stress test). The ER doctor checked his blood pressure frequently and found that it was gradually getting back to normal. However, the doctors were worried enough that our friend was admitted to the hospital for an overnight stay where he was attached to a monitor that continually displayed a perfectly normal pulse rate. He remained in bed until his blood pressure was back to normal, where it had been all of his life until he took the pills. He was seen and examined by an attending cardiologist, several residents, and some medical students. He was visited frequently during the night by the nurse on duty. He was finally discharged home the next morning in the very same physical condition that he was in when he went for his regular doctor's visit the previous day, but with bills from the exercise testing laboratory, the ambulance service, the cardiologists, and the hospital totaling several thousands of dollars.

In this case, the sensor was the doctor who took his own pulse, and if there is fault in what ensued, it was not the fault of the sensor. The point is that sensed information can drive action independent of the condition being sensed. The proliferation of sensors humming away around the clock will provide a lot of information that has the potential to better refine your care. The good doctor will relish that information, but also will know that her job is not to treat the numbers, but to care for the person providing the numbers. After all, people aren't easily reduced to numbers, and single-minded attempts to digitize them will not only keep health care from being as good as it can be but will also risk doing serious harm. *Beware the tyranny of sensors.*

THE DEEPER CONNECTION

Responding to a question during a Medscape interview, Malcolm Gladwell related what his eighty-five-year-old mother wants in a doctor. She wants "an individual physician who knows her well, who listens to her, whom she trusts and with whom she can periodically have extended conversations." Granted she is eighty-five and Canadian, but we suspect that most people want those things too. "I think it's about this deeper connection we all have to something important," Dr. Gawande says.

Even when each of us is fully wired with the latest sensors and has the complete sequence of our genome on a CD or in the cloud, there will still be a lot of uncertainties that affect our health and wellbeing. The good doctor understands that each of us is best cared for by using the carefully evaluated available evidence as a starting point, but interpreting that evidence in the context of the unique human being she is caring for. This doctor pays close attention to the experts and looks carefully at the numbers, recognizing that she needs all the help she can get to take the best care of you. But she does take care of *you*.

Perhaps for each branch point on the medical decision tree, there should be three options, yes, no, or maybe. If the options are honestly considered, the maybe branch will get the most traffic. If you are to avoid the tyranny of experts and sensors, you will have to cross the bridge of maybes that connects the hard data and confident expertise to the less certain world of human health and wellbeing. You will need a guide.

CHAPTER 17

The Hope for a Digitally Powered Doctor

Medical judgment can be taught . . . but it cannot be neatly handed
over as the occasion demands it. It is the irreplaceable and
untransferable contribution that the healer makes to the
suffering individual who would be healed.

—SHERWIN B. NULAND

If, as knowledgeable people claim, we teeter on the brink of
a digital cataclysm that will destroy medicine as we know it,
what will become of our good doctor? Will she morph into
University of California, San Francisco professor Robert
Wachter's *Digital Doctor*, doing medicine by the numbers, no
longer so interested in knowing you as a unique person? Will
the uncertainties evaporate in the heat and light of technological progress? Is this partnership concept we've tried so
hard to sell doomed to wind up in a decade or two on a trash
heap of anachronisms, relics of a predigital era that are no
longer relevant?

Well, it is quite certain that the world of health and medical care will look, feel, and be very different two decades
from now. Exactly how it will be different is impossible to
predict—too many unknown unknowns—but science, technology, and societal pressures are potent drivers of change.
Where that blend of necessity and potential will take us is

anybody's guess, but it will have to deal with human beings, imperfect as we are and capricious as we are capable of being.

THE DOCTOR AS HEALER

We humans cannot be reduced to numbers, and we have needs that cannot be fully digitized. Care of human disease has always involved a *healer*. That role addresses a fundamental human need that will still be integral to humanness two decades or even two millennia from now.

The doctor we've described in this book is a healer. What does that mean? In an effort to bring some rigor to the definition of *the art of medicine*, Larry Churchill and David Schenck at Vanderbilt's Center for Biomedical Ethics and Society interviewed fifty practitioners who were considered expert healers by their peers and looked for what their interactions with patients had in common. They found eight themes: do little things (small courtesies, congenial manner); take time and listen; be open; find something to like, to love; remove barriers; let the patient explain; share authority; and be committed and trustworthy. Although, as mentioned earlier, we would add *touching*, our good doctor passes the healer test with flying colors. And, as we have said elsewhere, there is plenty of evidence that patients of these healers do better because of that relationship.

There is no magic or mystery involved in modern healing. It is just that there is an element to healing that depends on how flesh-and-blood humans interact with each other. The value of the healer is a lot more than how she diagnoses illnesses and decides on therapies. No matter how those medical care transactions are accomplished, we will still need a healer.

SOME PREDICTABLE EFFECTS OF SCIENCE, TECHNOLOGY, AND SOCIETAL PRESSURES

We're not foolhardy enough to attempt to paint a detailed portrait of health and medical care two decades from now (although neither of us is likely to be around to have to defend it), but some generalities that will have a major effect on how you and your doctor relate can be pretty confidently predicted.

Social pressures, including economics, accessibility, disparities in quality, politics, and ethical issues will force organizational changes. It has been predicted that mergers of most major health systems will result in a few megasystems which serve populations large enough to support both usual and sophisticated medical care and the education of health professionals in the necessary spectrum of specialties. So our ideal doctor will likely be employed by an organization with its own culture, responsibilities, and reward system. This will almost certainly mean that she will be paid a more-or-less fixed salary that will likely be less (corrected for inflation) than she might be able to make in a current margin-driven practice. We predict, however, that the most successful health care organizations will recognize the human and the monetary value of this breed of doctor and will support and reward her appropriately.

The science and technology will radically change how data is obtained, stored, protected, and interpreted. The explosion of information about health and disease and the technology for dealing with that information will affect how the relationship between evidence based and personalized medicine affects care. We represented that relationship graphically earlier, plotting *flexibility* as a function of *uncertainty*. The adjacent figure reproduces that graph and adds implications for how health care might be done in a decade or two. The proliferation of wearable and other remote devices for measuring health related variables, increasingly sophisticated analytical strategies, the universal availability of information via the internet, the interpretive power of computer algorithms (Archimedes? Watson?), and the ubiquity of the cloud will shift many conditions to the left on the flexibility/uncertainty curve. Health care could look something like this:

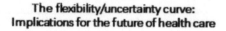

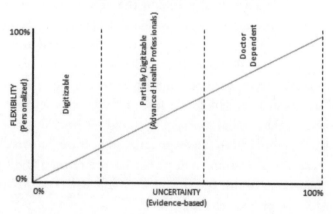

As more and more reliable general and personal information relevant to diagnosis and therapy of conditions accumulates, uncertainty will be reduced. That will decrease the need for the flexibility that is essential to adapting the evidence to an individual person. For a growing number of diagnoses and therapies, uncertainty will be reduced enough that *care can be digitized*, that is, done entirely electronically without any direct involvement of a health professional, with minimal risk of errors. Otitis media, an ear infection common in children, is a simple example. Your smart phone might have an attachment and an app that detects a red and bulging eardrum, impedance audiometry could indicate fluid in the middle ear, and an at-home simple test of samples of material from the ear canal would indicate the presence or absence of bacteria. Those data would be automatically entered into the appropriate website and you would be handed a diagnosis and a treatment plan. If the infection was bacterial, a prescription for the appropriate antibiotic would emerge from your printer or be sent electronically to your designated pharmacy. You'd make follow-up smart phone measurements every couple of days. The computer would keep you informed of your kid's progress and would let you know if something else needed to be done or would alert your doctor if things weren't going as expected. Such streamlining of the care of simple problems could save a lot of time and money.

Diagnosis and therapy of a large group of conditions will continue to be uncertain, but much less uncertain than now. Care of these disorders will be *partially digitizable*. The digital world can go a long way toward dealing with these conditions, but there is still too much uncertainty to turn the whole problem over to the computer. Some judgments will need to be made in the context of the specific patient, but those are judgments that can be reliably made by *advanced health professionals* trained specifically for that role. These professionals will be members of a health care team directed by a doctor who will be available when needed.

But treatment of some conditions will continue to be *doctor dependent*, that is, they will require the personal involvement of a doctor from the outset. These are maladies for which the diagnosis and treatment, in spite of our best efforts, continue to be very uncertain. Increasing information about and understanding of these conditions, coupled with a deeper understanding of each individual patient, will better the odds of success, but care will continue to require the hands-on involvement of a doctor.

Two decades hence, your genome will be fully sequenced and that information will be stored in your special nook in the cloud along with the rest of your −omic profile (proteome, metabolome, interactome, exposome, and maybe even microbiome). Your special cosmic nook will also house all of the other available information related to your health and wellbeing. This will include a reimagined and redesigned electronic medical record that will be a continually updated chronology of your health experience. The door to this information vault will be controlled by your thumbprint and will be inaccessible except with your permission. As science discovers more certain links between individual characteristics and health and disease, this deep knowledge of you and your life experiences will continually decrease the uncertainty in your care. But there will always be uncertainty. Human biology with all of its interrelationships is just too complex. The more we learn, the more we learn how much we don't know.

THE DIGITAL POWERED DOCTOR

So is there still a place for the healer in this technology-dense medical world of the future? We do not see the good doctor as competing with digitized health care, the hands-on physician pitted against the looming electronic juggernaut. On the contrary, we see this kind of doctor empowered by the digital world and, just as important, we see this doctor, the healer, as an indispensable complement to digital medicine, meeting a core human need that is not accessible electronically.

Digitization will give the doctor more time to heal. Delegating the care of straightforward clinical problems that currently consume large amounts of her time to computers and other health professionals will allow the doctor to focus more on nurturing a healing relationship with the patients for whom she cares. Efficient access to medical information and to individual patient data will make doctors better at their job, more confidently aware of who this patient is, what the problem is in that personal context, and what to do about it. Electronic systems that handle all of the clerical duties that will continue to be an essential part of medical practice will lift an enormous burden from doctors' shoulders. After all, that is what computers are supposed to be good at but haven't yet figured out how to do very well in a medical setting. Surely two decades is long enough to remedy that.

But what will be your personal doctor's role in this world of transformed medicine? First, she will be the professional whom you trust, who knows you, and who is committed to a partnership with you dedicated to keeping you healthy or getting you the best care when you are ill. She will be your reliable source of health information and advice. She will be available for you when you need her. She will be responsible for assuring that your diagnosis and therapy are correct when your condition falls in the full or partial digitization category, and if it turns out that you have been misassigned, this doctor will be there to straighten things out. When, in spite of everything, you are gravely ill or dying, she will hold your hand and likely weep with you and those who love you.

DESTRUCTION, DISRUPTION, OR EVOLUTION?

Probably all of the above. That is why we have limited our speculation to an outcome two decades hence and carefully avoided guessing much about the intervening process. Health care will be transformed, and transformation is seldom painless.

It seems likely that moving toward digital medicine will slaughter some of our sacred cows. The possibilities for radically different ways of getting and assimilating information may threaten traditional clinicians. They may also feel threatened by the emergence of new technology that seems to leave little space for the doctor in the patient-machine relationship. The need to become facile with computers will drive many doctors into retirement or another profession. The technology will disrupt both how medicine is done and how medical care is organized and supported. There will be false starts, blind alleys, mistaken directions taken, untenable promises made and then abandoned, and all of the other obstacles that rear up in the path of major change in a huge enterprise.

But, while there is an enormous health care industry, it is unlike other industries, which deal in goods and services less directly tied to the lives and wellbeing of every one of us. It is simply not imaginable that we will allow health care to go through a phase of total dysfunction, unable to provide essential care for those who need it. The profession cannot allow that to happen, and our broader society would be justly appalled at the thought of such a possibility.

So we predict that the *new medicine* will evolve, but without the orderliness that we usually expect of evolution. Some things we cherish will be destroyed, how we go about doing things will be disrupted, and the new health care paradigm will only gradually take on a form that works, although we cannot now imagine exactly what that form will be.

Time travel with us to an elite health care facility two decades into the future—it might well be that the only person we recognize there is the good doctor.

EPILOGUE

AN OPTIMIST'S DREAM

January 1, 2040

Well, thank heavens, at least I lived to see it. These last few years have been the most exhilarating of my long career practicing medicine. Who'd a thunk it? All that gloom and doom the pundits preached at the approach of the digital tsunami those decades ago were misguided. They underestimated the creativity and resilience of us humans when forced by circumstance and opportunity to reinvent what is arguably our most important social activity—caring for our health. For the last few years I have been a better doctor than ever before. I have come closer than I would ever have predicted to being the kind of professional that I dreamed of becoming back when I first realized that what I wanted was to do something with my head and hands that would help other people to be healthy and happy. Well, that's exactly what I've been doing lately and in my wildest dreams I would never have imagined that what has made it possible is the spectacular advances in science and technology that set me free to exploit the immense potential of my relationship with my patients to cure and to heal.

That's not to say that getting here was painless. It wasn't. Several times I came close to bailing out. Those courses in advanced computing took a personal toll, but I survived and even came to appreciate how much computer power could expand the possibilities. It was difficult to give up some control, especially to the inanimate world. That still bothers me. I still look over the computer's shoulder as it does its digital medicine thing. I'm still asking questions of almost everything. Adjusting my financial expectations was a little painful at first, but the rewards of escaping the escalating pressures for more "efficiency" from the managers and the chance to focus exclusively on the health and wellbeing of my patients more than compensate for a salary that doesn't quite match the old productivity based check. I still make a more than decent living. The managers seem surprised that the clinic makes plenty of money by forgetting about how long doctor visits take and paying more attention to how well the patients do. My patient visits take as long as they need to take to do the best possible job and that depends on who the person I'm seeing is and the nature of their problem—the time varies. I'm not at all surprised that this pays off for the managers.

My only regret is that I was ahead of my time. As dramatic as the changes I have been part of are, medicine is just beginning to realize the possibilities. I wish I had forty more years to hang around and watch my profession flourish. Of course if I did, I would have the same regret forty years from now. Change is the nature of this beast we call clinical medicine that we wrestle with every day and the only thing certain about it is that it will keep changing.

SOME OBSERVATIONS ON THE "NEW" MEDICINE

"May you live in interesting times," goes the Chinese curse. That's what practicing medicine these days seems like. The world of medicine is changing and the pace of change keeps ramping up. Much of the change is exhilarating—what we understand about human health is expanding and that opens new possibilities for helping people to be well and happy. That is, after all, why doctors do what they do, and the promises of new knowledge and technology that will help them do it better are exciting. In one way, we really look forward to the "New Medicine" that a lot of pundits are writing about these days.

In another way, we worry about where we are headed, worry that the powers that be will get carried away with the technology. If that means doing away with the human dimension of health and healing, then the two camps—science based and humanity based medicine—will be driven even further apart than they are now. Not good. And what really scares us is that the direction medicine takes may not be determined by the doctors and the patients whose interactions are the substance of health care. We worry that the potential of the technology and the inclinations of the health care "experts" (information specialists, people managers, systems designers, etc.) will jump the track leading to better health for more people and lead us into a system that fails to get the most out of the science by failing to recognize that health is essentially a flesh-and-blood human phenomenon.

The tragedy and the paradox that we may be courting is that dehumanizing health care, trusting the whole thing to gadgets and machines, would severely limit the potential of the science and technology. The real power of science and technology to make us healthier and happier is the power to enhance the critical functions of the doctor-patient partnership.

Whoever you people are out there making the crucial decisions about where medicine is going, please, for heaven's sake, involve some practicing doctors and real patients in the process!

There are reasons for hope. Our optimist's dream could actually come true. Some forward thinking medical schools aim to produce graduates who are, in the words of Clay Johnston, "the ones who are actually creating a system that's better for patients and for doctors."

NOTES

CHAPTER 1: THE DOCTOR YOU WANT (IT'S NOT WHO YOU THINK)

...**William Osler, the much revered godfather of modern American medicine** ... The William Osler Papers, "Father of Modern Medicine: The Johns Hopkins School of Medicine, 1889-1905," U. S. National Library of Medicine: Profiles in Science.

...**what Dr. Seuss calls** *the you that is You* ... Dr. Seuss, *Happy Birthday to You* (New York: Random House, 1959).

Michelle Roper (not her real name) knows, from personal experience ... Recollection of a patient encounter, KB.

...*listen to the patient he is telling you the diagnosis* ... William Bennett Bean, ed., *Sir William Osler: Aphorisms from His Bedside Teachings and Writings* (New York: Henry Schulman, Inc., 1950).

...*familial catamenial pneumothorax* ... J. Hinson, Jr., K. Brigham, and J. Daniell, "Catamenial Pneumothorax in Sisters," *Chest* 80, no. 5 (1981): 634-635.

CHAPTER 2: UNCERTAINTY IS ESSENTIAL TO PERSONAL HEALTH CARE

A middle-aged woman who worked as a laboratory technician ... Recollection of a patient encounter, KB.

...**Lewis Dahl concluded that a rice and fruit diet** ... Hema Bashyam, "Lewis Dahl and the Genetics of Salt-Induced Hypertension, *Journal of Experimental Medicine* 204, vol. 7 (2007): 1507.

...**Both low sodium intakes and high sodium intakes are associated with** *increased* **[emphasis added] mortality** ... N. Graudal, G. Jürgens, B. Baslund, and M.H. Alderman, "Compared with Usual Sodium Intake, Low- and Excessive-Sodium Diets Are Associated with Increased Mortality: A Meta-Analysis," *American Journal of Hypertension* 27 (1129): 1129-37.

. . . **Ancel Keys, a brilliant and charismatic nutritionist** . . . Roger Kaza, "Ancel Keys," *Engines of Our Ingenuity* 2469, http://uh.edu/engines/epi2469.htm.

. . . **published his results as a book in 1980** . . . Ancel Keys, ed., *Seven Countries: A Multivariate Analysis of Death and Coronary Heart Disease* (Cambridge: Harvard University Press, 1980).

. . . **analysis of data from over half a million people from 76 different studies** . . . Rajiv Chowdhury, MD, PhD; Samantha Warnakula, MPhil*; Setor Kunutsor, MD, MSt*; Francesca Crowe, PhD; Heather A. Ward, PhD; Laura Johnson, PhD; Oscar H. Franco, MD, PhD; Adam S. Butterworth, PhD; Nita G. Forouhi, MRCP, PhD; Simon G. Thompson, FMedSci; Kay-Tee Khaw, FMedSci; Dariush Mozaffarian, MD, DrPH; John Danesh, FRCP*; and Emanuele Di Angelantonio, MD, PhD*, "Association of Dietary, Circulating, and Supplement Fatty Acids with Coronary Risk: A Systematic Review and Meta-Analysis," *Annals of Internal Medicine* 160, vol. 6 (2014):398-406.

. . . **flyleaf of the Bible,** *interesting if true* . . . personal communication, to KB from James Hogg, MD.

. . . *The Median Isn't the Message* . . . Stephen Jay Gould, "The Median Isn't the Message," https://people.umass.edu/biep540w/pdf/Stephen%20Jay%20Gould.pdf.

About every six weeks over sixteen months a forty-four-year-old man . . . Susan Knight and Deborah Symmons, "Masterclass: A Man with Intermittent Fever and Arthralgia," *Annals of the Rheumatic Diseases* 57 (1998): 711-714.

Writing in the *New York Times***, Gina Kolata introduces us to one** . . . Gina Kolata, "Treatment for Leukemia, Glimpses of the Future," *The New York Times.* July 7, 2012, http://www.nytimes.com/2012/07/08/health/in-gene-sequencing-treatment-for-leukemia-glimpses-of-the-future.html?_r=0.

. . . **MATCH trial** . . . NCI-Molecular Analysis for Therapy Choice (NCI-MATCH) Trial. National Cancer institute. http://www.cancer.gov/about-cancer/treatment/clinical-trials/nci-supported/nci-match.

. . . *would revolutionize the diagnosis, prevention, and treatment of most, if not all, human diseases,* . . . Nicholas Wade, "A Decade Later, Genetic Map Yields Few New Cures," *The New York Times,* June 12, 2010.

. . . *a complete transformation in therapeutic medicine* . . . Nicholas Wade. "A Decade Later, Genetic Map Yields Few New Cures." *The New York Times,* June 12, 2010.

... John Murray complains in the *American Journal of Respiratory and Critical Care Medicine* that the definition of personalized medicine ... John Murray, "Personalized Medicine: Been There, Done That, Always Needs Work!," *American Journal of Respiratory and Critical Care Medicine* 185, no. 12 (2012): 1251-1252.

... Francis Collins calls the *Language of Life.* Francis Collins, *The Language of Life: DNA and the Revolution in Personalized Medicine* (New York: Harper Collins, 2010).

CHAPTER 3: FINDING YOUR DOCTOR: A FIELD GUIDE

In his book, *How Doctors Think*, Harvard physician Jerome Groopman ... Jerome Groopman, *How Doctors Think* (New York: Houghton Mifflin Company, 2007).

... *The ideal listener, it seems to me,* Copland writes ... Aaron Copland, "The Gifted Listener," *The Saturday Review*, pp. 41-44, September 27, 1952.

In his book, *The Black Swan*, ... Nassim Nicholas Taleb, *The Black Swan: The Impact of the Highly Improbable* (New York: Random House, 2007).

Christopher Chabris and Daniel Simmons made the video ... Christopher Chabris and Daniel Simons, *The Invisible Gorilla: And Other Ways Our Intuitions Deceive Us* (New York: Harmony, 2010).

... *When you hear hoof beats, think horses, not zebras,* ... "Zebra (Medicine)," Wikipedia, https://en.wikipedia.org/wiki/Zebra_(medicine).

... *In making the diagnosis of the cause of illness in an individual case, calculations of probability have no meaning* ... A.M. Harvey et al., *Differential Diagnosis*, 3rd ed. (Philadelphia: W. B. Saunders, 1979).

Nancy Pogue's (not her real name) personal experience is a good example ... "Zebras with Different Stripes: One Patient's Story," *SCOPE*, July 17, 2012.

Dr. Woodward's axiom is less and less relevant even to his specialty, infectious diseases, ... William Stauffer, MD, "Evolution of the Zebra: When You Hear Hoofbeats, You Need to Consider All Ungulates," *Minnesota Medicine*, November 2008.

... four sentences that mystery writer Louise Penny's fictional Montreal detective Armand Gamache ... Louise Penny's website, http://www.louisepenny.com/faqs.htm.

. . . **Press Ganey score of patient satisfaction** . . . http://www.pressganey.com/.

. . . **got bad scores because he refused to prescribe narcotics** . . . Richard Gunderman, "When Physicians' Careers Suffer Because They Refuse to Prescribe Narcotics," *The Atlantic*, October 30, 2013, http://www.theatlantic.com/health/archive/2013/10/when-physicians-careers-suffer-because-they-refuse-to-prescribe-narcotics/280995/.

. . . *the most satisfied patients are 12 percent more likely to be hospitalized and 26 percent more likely to die* . . . Joshua J. Fenton, MD, MPH; Anthony F. Jerant, MD; Klea D. Bertakis, MD, MPH; and Peter Franks, MD, "The Cost of Satisfaction: A National Study of Patient Satisfaction, Health Care Utilization, Expenditures, and Mortality," *Archives of Internal Medicine* 172 (2012): 405-411.

. . . *We can over-treat and over-prescribe. The patients will be happy, give us good ratings, yet be worse off* . . . William Sonnenberg, MD, "Patient Satisfaction Is Overrated," *Medscape*, March 6, 2014.

spaces in your togetherness . . . Kahlil Gibran, *The Prophet* (Eastford: Martino Fine Books, 2011).

CHAPTER 4: WHERE DOCTORS COME FROM

. . . **that really is why most people choose a medical career** . . . Danielle Ofri, MD, "Why Would Anyone Choose to Become a Doctor?," *The New York Times*, July 21, 2011.

. . . **psychologist Else Frenkel-Brunswik described aversion to ambiguity** . . . Else Frenkel-Brunswik, "Intolerance of Ambiguity as an Emotional and Perceptual Personality Variable," *Journal of Personality* 18 (1949): 2-143.

According to Johns Hopkins professor of medicine, Gail Geller, doctors with low tolerance for ambiguity . . . Gail Geller, ScD, "Tolerance for Ambiguity: An Ethics-Based Criterion for Medical Student Selection," *Academic Medicine* 88 (2013): 581-584.

. . . **recognized that medical students with high or low tolerance for ambiguity differ from each other in some important ways.** Gail Geller, Ruth R. Faden, and David M. Levine, "Tolerance for Ambiguity among Medical Students: Implications for Their Selection, Training and Practice," *Social Science & Medicine* 31 (1990): 619-624.

. . . validated scales for measuring how well one deals with ambiguity . . .
Gail Geller, Ruth R. Faden, and David M. Levine, "Tolerance for Ambiguity among
Medical Students: Implications for Their Selection, Training and Practice." *Social
Science & Medicine* 31 (1990): 619-624.

**. . . Massachusetts General Hospital (MGH) psychiatrist Helen Riess claims
that . . .** Bella English, "At MGH, Schooling Doctors in the Power of Empathy:
Center Draws Praise for a Basic Idea with Huge Effects," *Boston Globe,* August 16,
2015.

. . . some other specific things I can do to help make this relationship . . .
Susan Matthews, "10 Easy Ways to Improve Your Relationship with Your Doctor," *Everyday Health,* April 10, 2014, http://www.everydayhealth.com/news/easy-ways-im-
prove-relationship-with-doctor/.

Be clear and precise about the reason for your visit . . . "Patient Rights," UT
University Medical Group, http://www.utprimarycare.org/patient-rights/.

**. . . extrinsic (read money) and intrinsic (read feeling good about one's
work) motivations in affecting . . .** Timothy Judson, Kevin Volpp, and Allan
Detsky, "Harnessing the Right Combination of Extrinsic and Intrinsic Motivation
to Change Physician Behavior," *Journal of the American Medical Association* 314 (2015):
2233-2234.

In 2014, TEDMED convened . . . "Why Physicians Should Admit What They
Don't Know: TEDMED 2014, *AMA Wire,* Sepember 10, 2014, http://www.ama-as-
sn.org/ama/amawire/post/physicians-should-admit-dont-tedmed-2014.

Nothing in life is certain, **mused Ben Franklin,** *except death and taxes.* "Benjamin
Franklin Quotes," BrainyQuote, http://www.brainyquote.com/quotes/quotes/b/
benjaminfr129817.html.

There is no such uncertainty as a sure thing. "Robert Burns Quotes," BrainyQuote,
http://www.brainyquote.com/quotes/quotes/r/robertburn182938.html.

CHAPTER 5: THE YES–OR–NO OBSESSION

Sixty-six-year-old Hermione Barcrand (not her real name) . . . Recalled
patient encounter, KB.

The $50,000 Physical, Michael B. Rothberg, "A Piece of My Mind. The $50,000
Physical," *Journal of the American Medical Association* 311 (2014):2175-2176,
doi:10.1001/jama.2014.3415.

. . . *Choosing Wisely* **project that has created lists . . .** "Choosing Wisely: An Initiative of the ABIM Foundation," ABIM Foundation, http://www.choosingwisely. org/.

In 2009, just twelve medical tests deemed by expert review to have been done without an adequate indication cost . . . Michelle Andrews. "Doctors Estimate $6.8 Billion in Unnecessary Medical Tests." *The Washington Post*, October 31, 2011.

Nobody ever gets sued for ordering unnecessary tests, **. . .** Michelle Andrews. "$6.8 Billion Spent Yearly On Twelve Unnecessary Tests And Treatments," *Kaiser Health News,* October 31, 2011, http://khn.org/news/michelle-andrews-on-unnecce-sary-tests-and-treatments/.

Forty percent of men whose PSA measurement was equivocal, that is, *"provides no information about whether or not you have cancer,"* **. . .** Jamie Holmes. "Doctors Hate Ambiguity: How an Obsession with Certainty Can Hurt Patients' Health." From *Nonsense: The Power of Not Knowing* by Jamie Holmes. Crown, 2015.

. . . **Agency for Health Care Research and Quality suggests the following ten questions . . .** "The 10 Questions You Should Know: Questions Are the Answer," Agency for Health care Research and Quality, http://www.ahrq.gov/pa-tients-consumers/patient-involvement/ask-your-doctor/10questions.html.

CHAPTER 6: THE ILLUSION OF INFALLIBILITY

When Ms. Black discovered a golf ball size lump on her chest, . . . Trisha Torrey, "Trisha's Misdiagnosis Story." *Every Patients Advocate*, http://everypatientsadvo-cate.com/who-is-trisha/misdiagnosis/.

. . . *Infallibility refutes the possibility of error to which all human beings are suscep-tible. Authority is the uniform it wears.* Richard Hayward. "Balancing Certainty and Uncertainty in Clinical Medicine." *Developmental Medicine & Child Neurology* 48 (2006): 74–77.

A man getting chemotherapy in his small local hospital was responding . . . "My Friend's Story," The Fecal Translant Foundation: Patient Stories, September 23, 2014. http://thefecaltransplantfoundation.org/patient-stories/.

A nurse in a Washington hospital was alarmed when she saw that her patient . . . . Laurie Tarkan, "Arrogant, Abusive and Disruptive—and a Doctor," *The New York Times*, December 1, 2008.

A Washington pediatrician had practiced medicine for . . . Sandra G. Boodman, "Doctors' Diagnostic Errors Are Often Not Mentioned But Can Take A Serious Toll," *Kaiser Health News*, May 6, 2013.

In one survey 67 percent of health care workers at 102 nonprofit hospitals . . . Laurie Tarkan, "Arrogant, Abusive and Disruptive—and a Doctor," *The New York Times*, December 1, 2008.

An attending doctor flings a patient's chart clear across a nurses' station . . . personal recollection, KB.

***Institute for Safe Medication Practices* says that forty percent** . . . Laurie Tarkan, "Arrogant, Abusive and Disruptive—and a Doctor," *The New York Times*, December 1, 2008.

For example, there are guidelines that recommend giving a heart drug . . . Confidential personal communication to MMEJ.

A middle-aged professional acquaintance of ours . . . Personal recollection, KB.

. . . ***"never let the facts get in the way of truth."*** Farley Mowat, *Wikipedia* https://en.wikipedia.org/wiki/Farley_Mowat.

CHAPTER 7: THE "POOR ME" SYNDROME

In a survey of twelve thousand physicians only 6 percent described . . . Sandeep Jauhar, "Why Doctors Are Sick of Their Profession: American Physicians Are Increasingly Unhappy with Their Once-Vaunted Profession, and That Malaise Is Bad for Their Patients," *The Wall Street Journal*, August. 29, 2014, http://www.wsj.com/articles/the-u-s-s-ailing-medical-system-a-doctors-perspective-1409325361.

Sandeep Juahar, author of *Doctored*, . . . Sanjeep Juahar, *Doctored: The Disillusionment of an American Physician* (New York: Farrar, Straus and Giroux, 2014).

Fifty-eight percent of two thousand physicians surveyed . . . **Over one eight-year period the number of doctors** . . . Sandeep Jauhar, "Why Doctors Are Sick of Their Profession: American Physicians Are Increasingly Unhappy with Their Once-Vaunted Profession, and That Malaise Is Bad for Their Patients," *The Wall Street Journal*, August. 29, 2014, http://www.wsj.com/articles/the-u-s-s-ailing-medical-system-a-doctors-perspective-1409325361.

. . . **thousand-plus doctors questioned in 2009** . . . M. Quinn, A. Wilcox, E. J. Orav, D. W. Bates, and S. R. Simon, "The Relationship between Perceived Practice

Quality and Quality Improvement Activities and Physician Practice Dissatisfaction, Professional Isolation, and Work-Life Stress," *Medical Care* 47 (2009): 924-928.

. . . I used to be a doctor, now I'm a clerk . . . half of 7,200 doctors surveyed by the Mayo Clinic . . . Roni Caryn Rabin, "A Growing Number of Primary-Care Doctors Are Burning Out. How Does This Affect Patients? *The Washington Post*, March 31, 2014.

. . . half of practicing primary care physicians spend less than 16 minutes . . . Two thirds of primary care providers spend ten hours . . . Carol Peckham, "Medscape Physician Compensation Report 2015," *Medscape*, April 21, 2015.

. . . Abraham Verghese makes the point most elegantly in his TED talk . . . Abraham Verghese, "A Doctor's Touch," TED, http://www.ted.com/talks/abraham_verghese_a_doctor_s_touch.

All but 5 percent of the explosive growth in the health care workforce . . . Robert Kocher, "The Downside of Health Care Job Growth," *Harvard Business Review*, September 23, 2013.

. . . half of practicing doctors do not feel *fairly compensated* . . . the average annual salary of a primary care doctor was $195,000; for specialties . . . cumulative lifetime earnings were about $6.5 million for primary care doctors and more than $10 million for specialists. Carol Peckham, "Medscape Physician Compensation Report 2015," *Medscape*, April 21, 2015.

. . . median household annual income in the U.S. . . . Carmen DeNavas-Walt and Bernadette D. Proctor, "Income and Poverty in the United States: 2013: Current Population Reports," U.S Census Bureau, Department of Commerce, Economics and Statistics Administration, September, 2014.

. . . unpaid medical bills are the leading cause . . . Dan Mangan. "Medical Bills Are the Biggest Cause of U. S. Bankruptcies: Study," *CNBC*, June 25, 2013, http://www.cnbc.com/id/100840148.

Martin Karnovsky and Janis Finer . . . Roni Caryn Rabin, "A Growing Number of Primary-Care Doctors Are Burning Out. How Does This Affect Patients?," *The Washington Post*, March 31, 2014.

. . . Dr. Victoria Sweet at the Laguna Honda hospital . . . Victoria Sweet, "Should a Doctor Be Like a Gardener?," *The Wall Street Journal*, April 25, 2012.

. . . patients of high empathy doctors have 40 percent fewer severe complications of their diabetes . . . Meghan O'Rourke, "Doctors Tell All—and It's Bad," *The Atlantic*, November 2014.

. . . fifty thousand and two hundred thousand people die each year in American hospitals of preventable medical errors . . . *To Err Is Human: Building a Safer Health System*, Institute of Medicine (Washington, D. C.: The National Academies Press), https://doi.org/10.17226/9728.

. . . study of seven hundred surgeons who believed they had made a medical error . . . T. Shanafelt, C. Balch, G. Bechamps, T. Russell, L. Dyrbye, D. Satele, P. Collicott, P. Novotny, J. Sloan, and J. Freischlag, "Burnout and Medical Errors Among American surgeons," *Annals of Surgery* 251 (2010): 995-1000.

. . . conventional medicine, *kills more people than it saves*. . . . "New Report: Preventable Medical Mistakes Account for One Sixth of All Annual Deaths in the United States," *Mercola*, October 9, 2013, http://articles.mercola.com/sites/articles/archive/2013/10/09/preventable-medical-errors.aspx.

CHAPTER 8: THE DIFFERENCE BETWEEN "FACTS" AND FACTS

***Elementary, my dear Watson.* . . .** Karl Smallwood, "Sherlock Holmes Never Said "Elementary, My Dear Watson," *Today I Found Out*, August 27, 2013, http://www.todayifoundout.com/index.php/2013/08/sherlock-holmes-never-said-elementary-dear-watson/.

British gastroenterologist Andrew Wakefield and colleagues . . . "Times Topics: Andrew Wakefield," *The New York Times*, http://www.nytimes.com/topic/person/andrew-wakefield.

. . . *the holy text* of an anti-vaccine movement . . . "The Anti-vaccination Movement: A Study in Propaganda, Disinformation, and Dishonesty, *What Would Jack Do?*, February 3, 2015, http://whatwouldjackdo.net/2015/02/the-anti-vaccination-movement-a-study-in-propaganda-disinformation-and-dishonesty.html.

Something like this actually happened in 2015. "Measles Cases and Outbreaks," Centers for Disease Control and Prevention, http://www.cdc.gov/measles/cases-outbreaks.html.

. . . *absence of evidence is not evidence of absence* . . . "Carl Sagan Quotes," BrainyQuote, http://www.brainyquote.com/quotes/quotes/c/carlsagan589698.html.

Nassim Nicholas Taleb's fascinating book . . . Nassim Nicholas Taleb, *The Black Swan: The Impact of the Highly Improbable* (Random House Trade Paperbacks, 2010).

. . . Scottish doctor, Archibald Cochrane . . . Hriday Shah and Kevin Chung, "Archie Cochrane and His Vision for Evidence-Based Medicine," *Plastic and Reconstructive Surgery* 124 (2009): 982-988.

. . . *Effectiveness and Efficiency: Random Reflections on Health Services* . . . A. L. Cochrane, *Effectiveness and Efficiency: Random Reflections on Health Services* (London: Nuffield Provincial Hospitals Trust, 1973).

. . . the Cochrane Collaboration considers randomized controlled trials . . . A. Levin, "The Cochrane Collaboration," *Annals of Internal Medicine* 135 (2001): 309-312.

. . . 2010 *Atlantic* article titled, *Lies, Damned Lies and Medical Science* . . . David Freedman, "Lies, Damned Lies, and Medical Science," *The Atlantic*, November 2010.

. . . this has been called the *Hype Cycle* . . . "Hype Cycle," Wikipedia, https://en.wikipedia.org/wiki/Hype_cycle.

. . . observational studies that were subsequently tested . . . Stanley Young and Alan Karr, "Deming, Data, and Observational Studies: A Process Out of Control and Needing Fixing," *Significance,* pp. 116-120, September 2011.

. . . eponyms for these phenomena (Placebo effect, Hawthorne effect), we like *Pygmalion effect*. Stephen W. Draper, "The Hawthorne, Pygmalion, Placebo and Other Effects of Expectation: Some Notes," http://www.psy.gla.ac.uk/~steve/hawth.html.

. . . emerging field of *pragmatic research trials*. "Explanatory and Pragmatic Research," *Open Philanthropy Project*, http://www.openphilanthropy.org/explanatory-and-pragmatic-research.

CHAPTER 9: INFORMATION IS NOT NECESSARILY KNOWLEDGE

Paradoxically, the more I learn about . . . Phillip Peterson, *Get Inside Your Doctor's Head* (Baltimore: The Johns Hopkins University Press, 2013).

Dr. Rachel Moon, professor of pediatrics at the University of Virginia, an expert . . . M. Chung, R. Oden, B. Joyner, A. Sims, and R. Moon, "Safe Infant Sleep Recommendations on the Internet: Let's Google It," *Journal of Pediatrics* 161 (2012):1080-1084.

A Mayo Clinic study several years ago . . . F. North, W. Ward, P. Varkey, and S. Tulledge-Scheitel, "Should You Search the Internet for Information about Your Acute Symptom?," *Telemedicine Journal and E-Health* 18 (2012): 213-218.

Todd Rose, director of the Mind, Brain, and Education program at Harvard, uses . . . Todd Rose, *The End of Average* (San Francisco: HarperOne, 2015).

One study published in 2012, concludes that over forty thousand patients die annually in this country's intensive care units . . . Bradford Winters, Jason Custer, Samuel Galvagno Jr., Elizabeth Colantuoni, Shruti Kapoor, HeeWon Lee, Victoria Goode, Karen Robinson, Atul Nakhasi, Peter Pronovost, David Newman-Toker. "Systematic Review: Diagnostic Errors in the Intensive Care Unit: A Systematic Review of Autopsy Studies," *BMJ Quality & Safety* 10 (2012): 1136.

make publicly available . . . information on physician performance that provides comparable information on quality and patient experience measures . . . Section 10331(a) of the Patient Protection and Affordable Care Act (ACA).

. . . a web site called *Physician Compare* **. . .** Physician Compare Initiative, www.cms.gov/Medicare/Quality-Initiatives-Patient-Assessment-Instruments/physician-compare-initiative/Physician-Compare-Overview.html.

. . . before long, to monitor in real time, in quantitative terms . . . *more than thirty thousand new personal tracking projects are started by users every month.* **. . .** Gary Wolf, "The Data-Driven Life," *The New York Times Magazine,* April 28, 2010.

. . . will enable construction of my *quantified self* **. . .** Gary Wolf, "The Quantified Self," TED, https://www.ted.com/talks/gary_wolf_the_quantified_self?language=en.

American Heart Association's website encourages us to *Know Your Health Numbers* **. . .** "Know Your Health Numbers," American Heart Association, http://www.heart.org/HEARTORG/Conditions/Diabetes/PreventionTreatmentofDiabetes/Know-Your-Health-Numbers_UCM_313882_Article.jsp#.V9LSWZgrIhc.

. . . *value driven planning* **. . .** Matthew Leitch, "Value Driven versus Target Driven Planning," *Dynamic Management for an Uncertain World,* July 5, 2006.

CHAPTER 10: THE GOOD, THE BAD, AND THE UGLY OF STATISTICS

When we use single numbers to estimate uncertain future outcomes . . . Sam Savage, *The Flaw of Averages* (Hoboken: Wiley, 2009).

. . . *How to Lie With Statistics* . . . Darrell Huff, *How to Lie With Statistics* (New York: W. W. Norton and Company, 1993).

. . . **Presbyterian minister, Rev. Thomas Bayes** . . . "Thomas Bayes," Wikipedia, https://en.wikipedia.org/wiki/Thomas_Bayes.

An Essay towards solving a Problem in the Doctrine of Chances . . . Thomas Bayes, "An Essay Towards Solving a Problem in the Doctrine of Chances," *Philosophical Transactions of the Royal Society of London* 53 (1763): 370.

. . . **Kevin Boone uses the simple illustration of picking a probable winner of a two horse race** . . . Kevin Boone, "Bayesian Statistics for Dummies," http://www.kevinboone.net/bayes.html.

. . . **the Monty Hall problem** . . . F. D. Flam, " The Odds, Continually Updated," *The New York Times*, September 29, 2014, http://nyti.ms/Ylzkqv.

. . . **Phillip Peterson's ten rules for doctoring is** . . . Phillip K. Peterson, *Get Inside Your Doctor's Head* (Baltimore: Johns Hopkins University Press, 2015).

. . . **writer, Abigail Zuger, wonders whether such people are practicing medicine** . . . Abigail Zuger, MD, "Patient, Heal Thyself," *The New York Times*, January 5, 2015.

. . . **the *digitization of health care*** . . . Jessica Oaks, "The Digitization of Healthcare," *IT Briefcase: IT News Resources and Events*, July 7, 2015, http://www.itbriefcase.net/the-digitization-of-healthcare.

. . . **one approach is called *game theory*** . . . George Diamond, Alan Rozanski, and Michael Steuer. "Playing Doctor: Application of Game Theory to Medical Decision-Making," *Journal of Chronic Diseases* 39 (1986): 669-677.

Carolyn Tarrant and her associates at the University of Leicester . . . C. Tarrant, T. Stokes, and A. M. Colman, "Models of the Medical Consultation: Opportunities and Limitations of a Game Theory Perspective." *Quality and Safety in Health Care* 13 (2004): 461-466.

. . . **brainchild of Kaiser Permanente's David M. Eddy.** David Eddy and Leonard Schlessinger, "Archimedes: An Analytical Tool for Improving the Quality and Efficiency of Health Care," *NCBI Bookshelf*, http://www.ncbi.nlm.nih.gov/books/NBK22837/.

. . . **have called** *network medicine.* Albert-Laszlo Barabasi, Natalie Gulbahce, and Joseph Loscalzo, "Network Medicine: A Network-Based Approach to Human Disease," *Nature Reviews Genetics* 12 (2011): 56–58.

. . . **acquired by Evidera** . . . "Archimedes Has Been Acquired by Evidera: Expanding Modeling and Analytics Services and Providing Additional EvidencE-based Solutions for Our Customers," Evidera: Evidence Value Insight, http://archimedesmodel.com/.

. . . *The Median Isn't the Message* . . . Stephen Jay Gould, "The Median Isn't the Message," https://people.umass.edu/biep540w/pdf/Stephen%20Jay%20Gould.pdf.

CHAPTER 11: DON'T BELIEVE EVERYTHING YOU READ, NO MATTER WHERE YOU READ IT

. . . **didn't need this meme to convince** . . . "Don't Believe Everything You Read on the Internet Just Because There's a Picture with a Quote Next to It," http://weknowmemes.com/wp-content/uploads/2012/07/dont-believe-everything-you-see-on-the-internet.jpg.

Charles Fort published a work titled *The Book of the Damned* . . . Colin Bennett, *Politics of the Imagination: The Life, Work and Ideas of Charles Fort* (New York: Cosimo Books, 2010).

Retraction Watch, **which follows numbers of and reasons** . . . Ivan Oransky, "Weekend Reads: Gay Canvassing Study Saga Continues: Elsiever Policy Sparks Concern: A String of Scandals," Retraction Watch: Tracking Retractions as a Window into the Scientific Process, http://retractionwatch.com.

. . . **the very journals that your doctor ought to be able to trust** . . . Adam Marcus and Ivan Oransky, "What's behind Big Science Frauds?," *The New York Times*, May 22, 2015.

. . . **more likely to be published in a "high impact" journal; more likely to be cited** . . . Joseph L.Y. Liu, "The Role of the Funnel Plot in Detecting Publication and Related Biases in Meta-Analysis," *Evidence-Based Dentistry* 12 (2011): 121–122.

. . . *published results of scientific investigations are not* . . . T. D. Sterling, W. L. Rosenbaum, and J. T. Weinkam, "Publication Decisions Revisited: The Effect of the Outcome of Statistical Tests on the Decision to Publish and Vice Versa," *The American Statistician* 49 (1995): 108-112.

. . . obligates clinical investigators to post . . . Nicola Jones, "Half of U.S. Clinical Trials Go Unpublished: Results Are Reported More Thoroughly in Government Data Base Than in Journals," *Nature News and Comment*, December 13, 2013.

. . . Carolina Riveros and her colleagues searched that database . . . Carolina Riveros, Agnes Dechartres, Elodie Perrodeau, Romana Haneef, Isabelle Boutron, and Phillips Ravaud, "Timing and Completeness of Trial Results Posted at Clinicaltrials. gov and Published in Journals," *PLOS Medicine*, doi: 10:1371/journal.pmed 1001586.

. . . *The Lancet*, we, and the rest of the world, know now that the 1998 Lancet paper . . . "Andrew Wakefield," Wikipedia, http://en.wikipedia.org/wiki/ Andrew_Wakefield.

. . . The multistate measles epidemic in 2015 . . . Terrance McCoy, "The Disneyland Measles Outbreak and the Disgraced Doctor Who Whipped up Vaccination Fear," *The Washington Post Morning Mix*, January 23, 2015.

. . . *All Results Journals* (ARJournals) . . . "Negative Results Journals: A New Scientific Journal Publishes Negative Results," *Science News*, http://topsciencenews. blogspot.com/2010/11/negative-results-journals.html.

. . . *Journal of Negative Results in Biomedicine* . . . Gabriella Anderson, Haiko Sprot, and Bjrn R. Olsen, "Opinion: Publish Negative Results: Non-confirmatory or 'Negative' Results Are Not Worthless," *The Scientist News and Opinion*, January 15, 2013.

. . . recognize, out of a number of facts, which are incidental . . . "Sherlock Holmes' Top 10 Lessons for Problem Solvers," Young Associates Inc., http://www.youngassocinc.com/problemswesolve.html.

***Data! Data! Data!* Sherlock Holmes cried . . .** "Sherlock Holmes' Top 10 Lessons for Problem Solvers," Young Associates Inc., http://www.youngassocinc.com/problemswesolve.html.

. . . visionaries writing in *The Fourth Paradigm* . . . Tony Hey, Stewart Tansley, and Kristin Tolle, eds., *The Fourth Paradigm: Data-Intensive Scientific Discovery* (Redmond: Microsoft Research, 2000).

CHAPTER 12: MY STORY IS FRONT AND CENTER—NARRATIVE-BASED MEDICINE

Scientific thinking might be defined as learning to distinguish . . ." Paul Lee, "The Nature of Anecdotes," *Emner: Medical Quackery, Pseudoscience, Skepticism*, September 1, 2003, http://www.skepticreport.com/sr/?p=423.

Ms. Sydney Blasingame (not her real name) was ninety-eight years old . . .
Recollection of patient encounter, KB.

. . . three most dangerous words in a doctor's vocabulary . . . Harriet Hall,
"The Role of Experience in Science-Based Medicine," *Science-Based Medicine: Exploring Issues & Controversies in Science & Medicine,* April 12, 2011, https://www.science-basedmedicine.org/the-role-of-experience-in-science-based-medicine/.

Anecdotes about the location of food or mortal danger must have given some early humans an advantage . . . "The Plural of Anecdote is Not Data,"
Skeptical Medicine, May 25, 2014, https://sites.google.com/site/skepticalmedicine//the-plural-of-anecdote-is-not-data.

. . . claim it is: not based on facts; unscientific; often no more than a casual observation; and commonly just undocumented rumor. "Anecdotal Evidence," Wikipedia, http://wikipedia.org/wiki/Anecdotal_evidence.

. . . Chauvenet's criterion . . . "Chauvenet's Criterion," Statistics How To: Statistics for the Rest of Us, *http://www.statisticshowto.com/chauvenets-criterion/.*

. . . *narrative-based medicine* . . . Trisha Greenhalgh and Brian Hurwitz, eds., *Narrative Based Medicine,* 1st ed. (London: BMJ Books, 1998).

. . . *How Doctors Think*, Katherine Montgomery . . . Kathryn Montgomery, *How Doctors Think: Clinical Judgment and the Practice of Medicine,* 1st ed. (Oxford: Oxford University Press, 2005).

The point is elegantly made by David Watts in his *Perspective* article . . .
David Watts, "Perspective: Cure for the Common Cold," *New England Journal of Medicine* 367 (2012): 1184–1185.

. . . reflect on the meaning and implications of her experiences . . . David Hatem and Elizabeth A. Rider, "Sharing Stories: Narrative Medicine in an Evidence-Based World," *Patient Education and Counseling* 54 (2004): 251–253.

Alfred S. Reinhart was a Harvard medical student . . . Peter Tishler, "Soma Weiss, and Alfred S. Reinhart, and the care of the patient," *Perspectives in Biology and Medicine* 53, no. 1 (2010).

This is harder than I thought it would be . . . Kenneth Brigham, *Hard Bargain: Life-Lessons from Prostate Cancer . . . A Love Story* (New York: Harper House, 2001).

234 NOTES

... *the human encounter with the sick and desperate, the brave and dying, the healed and grateful* ... Philip Overby, "The Moral Education of Doctors," *The New Atlantis*, pp. 7-26, Fall 2005.

... **The Care of the Patient, Francis Peabody's classic** ... Francis Peabody, "The Care of the Patient," *Journal of the American Medical Association* 88 (1927): 877-882.

Writing about prior traumatic experiences boosted ... David Hatem and Elizabeth A. Rider, "Sharing Stories: Narrative Medicine in an Evidence-Based World," *Patient Education and Therapy* 54 (2004): 251-253.

British Medical Journal report says that less than one percent of patients ... Vera Kalitzkus and Peter Matthiessen, "Narative-Based Medicine: Potential, Pitfalls, and Practice, *Permanente Journal* 13 (2009): 80-86.

... *Journal of the American Medical Association*, **Jayshil Patel** ... Jayshil Patel, "Writing the Wrong," *Journal of the American Medical Association* 314 (2015): 671-672.

Solutions have been tried, including the use of a scribe ... Richard Byny, "The Tragedy of the Electronic Health Record," *The Pharos*, pp. 2-5, Summer 2015.

... *evidence-based medicine and the anecdote are uneasy bedfellows or an ideal couple?* Jilleen Kosko, Terry Klassen, Ted Bishop, and Lisa Hartling, "Evidence-Based Medicine and the Anecdote: Uneasy Bedfellows or Ideal Couple?," *Pediatrics Child Health* 11 (2006): 665-668.

CHAPTER 13: AN EXPERT ESCORT FROM GUIDELINES TO PROTOCOLS

Thirty-seven-year-old man, was admitted to the hospital with stomach pain, headache, vomiting ... Philippa Horsfield, Sanjay Deshpande, and Richard Ellis, "Killing with Kindness? Drug Reaction Eosinophilia with Systemic Symptoms (Dress) Masquerading as Acute Severe Sepsis," *Journal of Antimicrobial Chemotherapy* 64 (2009): 663-665.

... **guidelines from the Cochrane Collaboration, the American Pain Society** ... "Epidural Steroid Injections for Back Pain: Worth a Shot, or Should You Skip It?," *Consumer Reports*, March 2011.

... **Cochrane review adds the caveat** ... J. B. Staal, R. de Bie, H.C. de Vet, J. Hildebrandt, and P. Nelemans, "Injection Therapy for Subacute and Chronic Low-Back Pain," *Cochrane Database of Systematic Reviews*, July 16, 2008, doi: 10.1002/14651858. CD001824.pub3.

. . . nine million times every year in this country, a steroid is injected . . .
Pat Anson, "Study Questions Use of Steroids in Spinal Shots," *National Pain Report: Pain Medication*, September 18, 2013, http://nationalpainreport.com/study-questions-use-steroids-spinal-shots-8821712.html.

An infectious disease specialist had been puzzling over her patient . . .
Denise Grady, "Meningitis Cases Are Linked to Steroid Injections in Spine," *The New York Times Health*, October 2, 2012.

Cynthia Scribe's (not her real name) friends described her . . . "Child Care Worker among Five Killed in Meningitis Outbreak Traced to Routine Back Pain Injections at Hospital . . . Amid Fears Thousands at Risk across 23 States," *Daily Mail*, October 4, 2012.

. . . produced by New England Compounding Center . . . meningitis epidemic spread to 19 states . . . "New England Compounding Center Meningitis Outbreak," Wikipedia, https://en.wikipedia.org/wiki/New_England_Compounding_Center_meningitis_outbreak.

They reviewed around 1,800 stories from a dozen or more reputable . . .
Gary Schwitzer, "Addressing Tensions When Popular Media and Evidence-Based Care Collide," *BMC Medical Informatics and Decision Making* 13, suppl. 3 (2013): S3, doi: 10.1186/1472-6947-13-S3-S3.

CHAPTER 14: THE BENEFITS OF IGNORANCE

Real knowledge is to know the extent of one's ignorance. "Confucius Quotes," Brainy-Quote, http://www.brainyquote.com/quotes/quotes/c/confucius101037.html.

. . . *a good question is worth a lot more than a mediocre fact,* . . . "Quotes and Anecdotes," MA310, University of Kentucky, Spring 2001, http://www.ms.uky.edu/~lee/ma310sp01/anec.pdf.

Leonard Thompson's family doctor knew he had diabetes . . . Howard Markel, "How a Boy Became the First to Beat Back Diabetes, *PBS NEWSHOUR*, January 11, 2013, http://www.pbs.org/newshour/rundown/how-a-dying-boy-became-the-first-to-beat-diabetes/.

. . . Frederick Banting, a little known Toronto orthopaedic surgeon . . .
"The Discovery of Insulin," *Nobelprize.org*, http://www.nobelprize.org/educational/medicine/insulin/discovery-insulin.html.

University of Colorado surgeon Ben Eisman and his colleagues may have known . . . Claran Kelly, "Fecal Microbiota Transplantation—an Old Therapy Comes of Age," *New England Journal of Medicine* 368 (2012): 474-475.

Ms. Cawthon developed a persistent intestinal infection with *C. diff* that caused chronic debilitating diarrhea . . . Maryn McKenna, "Swapping Germs: Should Fecal Transplants Become Routine for Debilitating Diarrhea?" *Scientific American,* December 2011.

. . . randomized study published in the *New England Journal of Medicine* . . . Els van Nood, Anne Vrieze, Max Nieuwdorp, et al., "Duodenal Infusion of Donor Feces for Recurrent *Clostridium Difficile*," *New England Journal of Medicine* 368 (2013): 407-415.

. . . Stan Cohen's careful scrutiny of something simple that he didn't expect wound up changing . . . Adam Navis, "Epidermal Growth Factor," *The Embryo Project Encyclopedia,* http://embryo.asu.edu/pages/epidermal-growth-factor.

. . . major implications for cancer biology . . . John Mendelsohn, "Targeting the Epidermal Growth Factor Receptor for Cancer Therapy," *Journal of Clinical Oncology* 20, suppl. 1 (2002): 1-13.

. . . 1986 Nobel Prize in Physiology or Medicine . . . Stanley Cohen, "Nobel Lecture—Epidermal Growth Factor," *Bioscience Reports* 6 (1986): 1017-1028, 1086.

Stuart Firestein's fascinating little book, *Ignorance: How it Drives Science* . . . Stuart Firestein, *Ignorance: How it Drives Science* (Oxford: Oxford University Press, 2012).

Professor of Family Medicine Christy Ledford and colleagues surveyed . . . Christy Ledford, Dean Seehusen, Alexander Chessman, and Navkrian Shokar, "How We Teach Us Medical Students to Negotiate Uncertainty in Clinical Care: A Cera Study," *Family Medicine* 47 (2015): 31-36.

CHAPTER 15: THE LAYING ON OF HANDS

It is believed by experienced doctors that the heat which oozes . . . "Hippocrates and the Laying on of Hands," *The International Center for Reiki Training,* December 28, 2001, https://www.reiki.org/articles/hippocrates-and-laying-hands

. . . Roman DeSanctis jokingly lamented, . . . *if you come to our* . . . Richard Knox, "The Fading Art of the Physical Exam," *NPR Morning Edition,* September 20, 2010, http://www.npr.org/templates/story/story.php?storyId=129931999.

. . . **Sandeep Jauhar recounts his father's experience** . . . Sandeep Jauhar, "The Decline of the Physical Exam in Modern Medicine," *Pacific Standard*, July 2, 2014, https://psmag.com/the-decline-of-the-physical-exam-in-modern-medicine-ba64c8d8bd4b#.irdubkcv1.

. . . **Abraham Verghese, says,** *When one individual (a patient) seeks help from another individual* . . . Richard Knox, "The Fading Art of the Physical Exam," *NPR Morning Edition*, September 20, 2010, http://www.npr.org/templates/story/story.php?storyId=129931999.

. . . **writer Malcolm Gladwell says,** *What doctors and patients need is more time, not more technology.* Eric Topol, "Malcolm Gladwell: Future Docs Need More Time, Not Technology," *Medscape*, August 15, 2015, http://www.medscape.com/viewarticle/847711.

CHAPTER 16: THE FEAR OF A TYRANNY OF EXPERTS AND SENSORS

I worry that we could become tyrannized by a combination of experts and sensors . . . Bob Wachter, "My Interview with Atul Gawande," *Wachter's World*, January 6, 2015, http://community.the-hospitalist.org/2015/01/06/my-interview-with-atul-gawande/.

In a hospital where a certain general surgeon practiced . . . Jeffrey Parks, "How Algorithm Driven Medicine Can Affect Patient Care," *KevinMD.com*, January 30, 2012, http://www.kevinmd.com/blog/2012/01/algorithm-driven-medicine-affect-patient-care.html.

A foolish consistency, **Ralph Waldo Emerson** . . . Ralph Waldo Emerson, "Quotes," Goodreads, http://www.goodreads.com/quotes/353571-a-foolish-consistency-is-the-hobgoblin-of-little-minds-adored.

. . . **evidence based medicine began in the 1960s** . . . David Eddy, "The Origins of Evidence-Based Medicine—a Personal Perspective," *Virtual Mentor* 13 (2011): 55-60.

The National Guideline Clearinghouse maintains a database . . . Dan Mendelson and Tanisha Carino, "Evidence-Based medicine in the United States—De rigeur or Dream Deferred?," *Health Affairs* 24 (2005): 133-136.

. . . **Truman longed for a one handed economist** . . . Paul Krugman, *The Economist*, November 13, 2003.

Evidenced based medicine is maligned as, . . . *inconsistent with modern science, theoretically unsound* . . . Stephen Hicke, Andrew Hickey, and Leonardo Noriega, "The Failure of Evidence-Based Medicine?," *European Journal for Person Centered Health Care* 1 (2012): 69-79.

. . . that nothing is ever completely settled, that all knowledge is just probable knowledge. Atul Gawande, "The Mistrust of Science," *The New Yorker,* June 10, 2016.

Would you believe *Moonshot Medicine?* Martin LaMonica, "How the Google X Moonshot Idea Factory Works," *Xconomy.com*, September 23, 2014, http://www.xconomy. com/san-francisco/2014/09/23/how-the-google-x-moonshot-idea-factory-works/#.

. . . new moonshot project, the human body . . . Alistair Barr. "Google's New Moonshot Project: The Human Body." *The Wall Street Journal,* July 27, 2014.

. . . convince a million Americans to wear some sensors . . . Jocelyn Kaiser. "NIH Plots Million-Person Megastudy," *Science* 347 (2015): 817.

. . . creative destruction of medicine . . . *is ready to go* . . . Eric Topol. *The Creative Destruction of Medicine: How the Digital Revolution Will Create Better Health Care* (New York: Basic Books, 2013).

A seventy-five-year-old physician we know . . . Personal information, KB and MMEJ.

. . . Malcolm Gladwell related what his eighty-five-year-old mother wants in a doctor. Eric Topol, "Malcolm Gladwell: Future Docs Need More Time, Not Technology," *Medscape,* August 18, 2015, http://www.medscape.com/viewarticle/847711.

CHAPTER 17: THE HOPE FOR A DIGITALLY POWERED DOCTOR

Medical judgment can be taught . . . but it cannot . . . "Sherwin B. Nuland Quotes," BrainyQuote, http://www.brainyquote.com/quotes/authors/s/sherwin_b_nuland.html.

. . . Robert Wachter's *Digital Doctor* . . . Robert Wachter, *The Digital Doctor: Hope, Hype, and Harm at the Dawn of Medicine's Computer Age* (New York: McGraw Hill, 2015).

. . . rigor to the definition of *the art of medicine* . . . Larry R. Churchill, PhD, and David Schenck, PhD, "Healing Skills for Medical Practice," *Annals of Internal Medicine* 149 (2008): 720–724.

EPILOGUE

. . . in the words of Clay Johnston, . . . the ones who are actually creating . . . Sean Price, "UT-Austin Medical School's Curriculum Isn't Designed Just to Train Doctors—It's Built to Revolutionize Medicine," *Journal of Texas Medicine* 113, no. 5 (2017): 28–33.